W9-ARV-093

THE INDEPENDENT PRACTITIONER

**Practice Management for
the Allied Health Professional**

THE INDEPENDENT PRACTITIONER

**Practice Management for
the Allied Health Professional**

Robert M. Pressman
Rodie Siegler

The Dorsey Press
Homewood, Illinois 60430

© Robert M. Pressman and Rodie Siegler, 1983

All rights reserved. No part of this publication may be
reproduced, stored in a retrieval system, or transmitted,
in any form or by any means, electronic, mechanical,
photocopying, recording, or otherwise, without the prior
written permission of the copyright holder.

This publication is designed to provide accurate and
authoritative information in regard to the subject matter
covered. It is sold with the understanding that the
publisher is not engaged in rendering legal, accounting, or
other professional service. If legal advice or other expert
assistance is required, the services of a competent
professional person should be sought.

*From a Declaration of Principles jointly adopted by a Committee
of the American Bar Association and a Committee of Publishers.*

ISBN 0-87094-315-4

Library of Congress Catalog Card No. 82-73633

Printed in the United States of America

2 3 4 5 6 7 8 9 0 K 0 9 8 7 6 5

For Jonathan, Rebecca, Sarah and Stephanie

R.M.P.

Preface

What is the lure of private practice in the allied health professions? For some it is the money and the prestige. For others it is being able to help people in the most direct way possible by relieving them of pain and curing them of sickness. But surely, for most health professionals it is the course of action taken to guarantee that training will result in financial security and prestige while at the same time doing good for humanity. And such has been the case for the last 50 years or more.

Today it is less certain that those in the private delivery of health services can count on a guaranteed income in the upper brackets and a prestigious position in society. Instead of the proverbial doctor shortage, there are now murmurings of a doctor glut. Medical schools are currently graduating two doctors for every doctor who retires or dies (Reinhold, 1982). The most startling result is that the heavily urbanized profession of physician seems to be returning once again to the horse and buggy days of the country practice.

No longer are there scores of small cities and towns begging for doctors. In Morrisville, Vermont, for example, a town of little more than 2,000 people, there are more than two dozen doctors, 16 of them with specialties. Although Morrisville serves as a medical center for about 22,000 people in the surrounding area, Vermont is one of the poorer states in the union and the winters are long and hard. The assumption would be that northern Vermont would be one of the last places that would attract health professionals. However, Morrisville, Vermont is not an exception but an example of a recent trend in the distribution of doctors. Now, few towns are without access to a doctor and small cities of 20,000 people can often boast of a urologist, an opthalmologist, an orthopedist, and other of the more arcane specialties. If a small town is lacking in health professionals, it is not usually because of its size or location but because of such factors as a lack of medical insurance or other financial support for the health professions.

Other consequences of the end of the doctor shortage are a change in the economics of private practice. According to a 1982 study by the American Medical Association (cited in Reinhold, 1982), the average income of doctors in 1970 dollars, adjusted for inflation, has dropped from $40,000 in 1970 to

$38,000 in 1980. Office visits have dropped 10 percent, probably reflecting a greater reliance on the hospital emergency room for medical care. The number of doctors in group practice sharing the overhead has more than doubled since 1969, although that may not necessarily reflect economic factors so much as a change in philosophy and lifestyle. Another indicator is the number of doctors in the population: 194 per 100,000 in 1980 as compared to 152 in 1970.

What are the implications of a doctor glut for a young health professional with plans for opening a practice? More than ever, a private practice must be regarded as a business. Like the local retail shop or building contractor, there is no room any more for sloppy business practices. Where you decide to practice, the impression you make in the community, the quality of the service you offer, the manner in which you deal with people—all will have a bearing on how well you will do against the competition. How you manage your business—keeping careful records, keeping expenses down, collecting money owed for services, handling your employees—these may make the difference between making and losing money just as it does for any independent businessperson.

For those in related health professions, the doctor glut may have differing consequences. If the glut continues in the direction of more and more specialists, there may be more of a demand for the nurse practitioner, a person familiar with the medical profession, to guide the layperson through the labyrinth of medical care and handle the more mundane but very real illnesses that beset people, particularly the very young and the very old. For registered nurses, there will be more opportunities as doctors throng into the smaller communities and establish medical care centers. For other specialists, such as optometrists and neurologists, as small towns develop medical facilities, there should be an expansion of opportunities. With all this increased competition, there will be one important consequence that can easily be prophesied—better care will be provided for a greater number of people.

For the young health practitioner ready to open a practice, the message is clear. There may not be a pot of gold at the end of the rainbow, but there will be a good life. You will be your own boss, make your own decisions, order your own work life. For those who have been in practice for 5 or 10 years, this may be a good time to look at changes in business demands, to keep up with the competition and changing times.

This book was written to help with the decisions concerning the business aspects of private practice. Practice your healing arts to the best of your ability, but be alert to the business details. Above all, make the patient the primary focus of your efforts. Treat patients as well as you can clinically and at the same time handle them with care, as the business customers that they are. They will respect you for your professionalism in both of those important aspects of a private practice.

Robert M. Pressman
Rodie Siegler

Acknowledgments

A number of people provided assistance in the preparation of this book. We would like to acknowledge their participation: Susan E. Whitney, Office Manager; Deborah B. Brennan, Library Director, North Kingstown Free Library; Timothy P. Jackson, Safeguard Business Systems; Denise Akey, Gale Research Company; Jeremiah O'Connell, M.D.; Lyman A. Davenport, M.D.; Burt A. Jordan, D.D.S.; Albert E. Carlotti, Jr., D.D.S. We would also like to acknowledge the assistance of the following companies and organizations: American Psychological Association; American Psychiatric Association; American Dental Association; National Association of Social Workers; B.M.A. Audio Cassettes; Thought Technology, Ltd.; Safeguard Business Systems; Newport Hospital Medical Library; South County Hospital Medical Library; Psychotherapy Finances; and Medical Economics, Inc.

Contents

1

Private practice

PRIVATE PRACTICE VERSUS INSTITUTIONAL PRACTICE

Health practitioners, perhaps more than any other working people, will find an ambivalence—a continuous dilemma—in their motivating factors toward work. We work to earn a living; that is, we work to make money. Businesspeople feel perfectly justified in adding a percentage for their profit. Making a profit is not only a right of a business but an obligation. If you don't make money, what are you doing running a business? Health practitioners, on the other hand, have an obligation first and foremost to their patients. Theirs are helping professions. If they don't help their patients, what are they doing practicing their profession? Indeed, there is a resentment today toward the wealth that some of the conspicuously rich private health professionals manage to accumulate. The message from society seems to be that it is fair for businesspeople to make money, but not fair for health practitioners. This is the dilemma that each private health professional must look at squarely when deciding to go into private practice.

Private practice consists of two important factors, each carrying equal weight. One is the delivery of health care. The other is the operation of a successful, profitable business. Each depends on the other for its success. A health practitioner in charge of a private practice must be equally knowledgeable about both the health care he or she is dispensing to patients and the management of a business. Health practitioners may spend years in school and in the various forms of supervised practice without ever encountering the exchange of money for services that characterizes private practice. As students they are never instructed in accounting, banking, real estate, building codes, insurance, personnel practices, and all the business-related details encountered in making a living from the practice of their profession. They are dumped out of school full of confidence in their ability to help people to regain or keep their health and confident in the knowledge that they have trained themselves in a profession that will in some arcane way result in a high standard of living. For many, learning to run their practice as a business involves many more years of study and many mistakes.

The alternative to private practice is working for someone else, if not in a group practice then in an institutional setting. Before making the final decision to open a private practice, some thought should be given to working as a professional in an institution. A discussion of the advantages and disadvantages of private versus institutional practice follows.

A young woman graduated from a Ph.D. program in clinical psychology. She was wise in the ways of institutions, having promoted institutional funds for both her master's degree and her doctorate. Throughout those lean years in graduate school she held on to the notion that at the end of the tunnel there would be enough money to buy some of the nicer things in life, such as a decent place to live, some new clothes, and a new car. Clutching her diploma in hand, she found that after 20 years in an institutional setting (school), an environment in which she felt self-confident and could do good work, she was suddenly at a loss. Her father suggested the navy. She was promised interesting work (a chance to work with the women at the Naval Academy), a good salary, a better than starting officer's rank—in short, a well-defined place in society—and she grabbed the offer. She felt more comfortable manipulating her career within an institution than coping as an independent practitioner out on her own. What are some of the factors that set private practice apart from a practice in an institutional setting?

Some definitions

In private practice there is a contract freely entered into between the health practitioner and the client/patient: the practitioner delivers health care; the patient pays a fee directly to the practitioner for that care. The health practitioner in most cases maintains an office—a business setting in which health care is delivered.

A private practice has all the characteristics of a business including the profit motive. It has a location; it delivers a service; it pays taxes; it may be subject to liability; it may have employees who must be paid and supervised; it must make money or close its doors and therefore is subject to record-keeping and accounting practices; and its activities must be cost efficient.

In an institution, on the other hand, the contract is between the practitioner and the institution: the practitioner will deliver health services to those patients for which the institution has made itself responsible; the institution will pay the practitioner; provide a setting (an office and equipment); but all contact with the patient other than the delivery of health care will be the responsibility of the institution. The practitioner may be compensated per patient, per hour, be paid a salary, work part time or full time.

An institutional setting may take many forms. The government is a major employer of health practitioners at the local as well as the federal level. The armed forces, including veteran facilities, employ health practitioners to deliver health care in hospitals as well as to work in administrative positions. At the local level, health professionals are employed in hospitals, clinics, mental institutions, and schools. Private industry may be a likely employer for a nurse, mental health practitioner, or a doctor. Nonprofit institutions, in addition to hospitals, include mental health clinics and residences, visiting nurse associations, schools and universities, and all the private research institutions. Generally in these institutional settings, the health professional exercises only his or her expertise in health care. The institution maintains the administrative functions.

Advantages of private practice

Perhaps in defining private versus institutional practices, the institutional practice sounds more desirable. Practitioners can devote their energies and their time to patients. They do not have to have any talents for administrative detail. They take no business risks. Why then do the great majority of health professionals choose to work on their own?

Money. The major incentive is money. The potential for making more money, and the possibility of making a lot more money, lies in a private practice. There is a limit to institutional salaries. Further, the salary range is known. This range is high enough to attract quality professionals, but more money can be made outside the institution.

The private practitioner is able to determine his or her own rate structure. This is an essential key to making money. If inflation continues at a two-digit rate, private practitioners can increase their fees and adjust their incomes to the inflation rate—a flexibility not often afforded in an institutional practice.

Being your own boss. For most people, the second most important incentive is to be one's own boss or to work in a partnership with a few respected colleagues. Traditionally, the health practitioner has had an independent status. In private practice one is not subject to the constraints of institutional rules and administrative arrangements not of one's own making. Working under the supervision of those above in a hierarchy is not comfortable for many professional people. You may not agree with certain clinical decisions that are made in an institutional setting. You, quite frankly, may not like the way a place is managed. And, one might say, that just as it is a part of most people's ambitions to own their own house, it is the American dream to be in business for oneself. Health practitioners are particularly susceptible to such a philosophy.

Work constraints. In an institutional setting you are hired to dispense health care within certain limited parameters. You may be hired, for example, as a pediatric nurse in a county hospital. After seven or eight years you find yourself more interested in the adolescents you see than the babies. You earn a master's degree in counseling with a view to working with teenagers. But your slot at the hospital gives you no scope to grow professionally. You are a good pediatric nurse, especially conscientious with the premature babies and they are not willing to replace you. You can go into private practice or you can find another job that will include counseling adolescents. One staff psychologist asked for time and expenses to go to a seminar on family therapy. He was refused on the basis that they already had a family therapist and had no need of such expertise on his part. Institutions are not usually flexible enough to encourage individual growth.

Time management. In private practice your time is your own. You can take Fridays off (as many dentists do) or take the whole month of August, the traditional vacation time for psychoanalysts. You can see patients only in the afternoon or be on call 24 hours a day. As you get older you can slow down and see patients only a couple of times a week, if you wish. You can go to meetings or take time to come home for lunch to see your new baby. You keep control over your own schedule and thereby your own life.

Diversity and personal growth. You can expand your areas of expertise when you are on your own in private practice. One physician trained as a pediatrician. He moved into child psychiatry after extensive training in psychoanalysis. His interests then narrowed to the emotional problems of chronically sick and dying children, at this point combining his private practice with a hospital staff position. As a result of seeing the effect of television on the children in his hospital, he became an expert on television violence. He introduced a closed TV circuit into his hospital and then sought expertise in television production in order to establish first-rate programming using the hospital TV equipment. This doctor started out as a private practitioner and from this vantage point was able to control the scope of his work in the institutional setting. Topnotch researchers can also dictate to their institution. They write their own grants and bring in their own money. But for the average medical professional, the institution is more limiting. For the most part professionals maintain a greater control over the work they do in private practice than in an institutional setting.

Patient population.   Private practitioners, except in medicare and medicaid mills, tend to treat middle-class patients. Most practitioners are more comfortable in the more familiar social interaction with middle-class people. Middle-class people tend to be more self-sufficient and easier to manage. They honor their appointments, take their pills, and follow directions. A poor person, for example, is apt to call at the last minute, if at all, to say the car broke down—and it has, in fact, broken down. For the poor, life is more complicated; they are more often victimized. For the practitioner working with the poor, providing continuity in health care may be more difficult and frustrating. The poor may have multiple health problems because of poor nutrition, poor housing, extreme emotional problems—all the ills associated with a lack of money in our society. In institutional settings, the poor tend to be the majority in the patient population.

Prestige.   Except for certain major research institutions, there is more prestige accorded to medical practitioners who work for themselves. And rightly so. Although in prestigious institutions researchers are honored for their own work, in other lesser institutions the practitioner is to a large extent channeled into a narrow work life. In a rough and ready way, prestige follows and is awarded for innovation and independence.

Disadvantages of private practice

Risk.   The principal disadvantage of private practice is that there is no guarantee that the money will come in. This is a major risk—a risk you share with every person who runs a business. First you must establish yourself in the community. This takes time during which you have to support yourself when your appointment book is not filled. Most important—attracting patients to your office door depends on your own efforts, as does keeping a steady stream of them coming each year.

Salary versus fees. In private practice you make money only when you are actually providing health care to a patient. That means that telephone time cannot be charged out. Lunch, journal-reading to keep up with your specialty, talking to colleagues for purposes of referral or second opinions, record-keeping, writing, and research (unless you have been accepted for a grant) are all done on your own time. You don't get paid when you are on vacation or are sick. In an institution you get your salary, in a sense, for just being there. And you get paid even when you are not there as, for example, if you are sick or on holiday, or attending professional meetings. A private practitioner cannot afford to be sick and although you have the freedom to take vacations, you may not do so because of the pressure and your feeling of responsibility for your patients.

Business management. In private practice you must learn to be a business manager. You will bear the responsibility for business decisions and, furthermore, you will have to take the time out of your clinical work for running your practice as a business. For example, you will have to choose a location for your office and rent it, hire and fire personnel, choose an accountant and/or a lawyer whom you can trust, become knowledgeable about taxes, investments, borrowing, buying services, and dealing with salespeople. The major thrust of this book is to help you to cope with business decisions.

Responsibility for patients. In private practice you have the prime responsibility for the health of patients who entrust themselves to you. The weight of making decisions crucial to other people's lives, is on you. Their money will be spent, if they do not have insurance, and their time. They may suffer pain, both real and psychic, because of you. The private practitioner can cause a great deal of unpleasantness for a patient. The legal responsibility for patients' well-being falls into the category of malpractice. A malpractice suit may be brought against a private practitioner for unnecessary harm to a patient. (See Chapter 8 for a discussion of malpractice.)

The other side of the coin, of course, is the knowledge that you have been able to help a patient. In private practice you have the satisfaction of following a patient's progress and if you practice in a neighborhood setting, of knowing and serving the same families over the years. And for many private practitioners, therein lies one of the greatest rewards of working in the health professions.

Interaction with patients and their families over the years is also helpful in weighing alternative treatments. Knowing patients and their circumstances is an important clue in assessing medically and psychologically the best way to treat them as well as being able to do the necessary follow-up work. So that responsibility cuts two ways—as an awesome personal burden and as an advantage in treatment.

Isolation. Many private practitioners find private practice isolating. It may be a strain, especially for mental health practitioners who see only a limited number of patients, and those, week after week. There is no one to share patient problems with. There are no serendipitous encounters with colleagues in which to exchange the gossip of the profession, give and take advice, or even to seek referrals. Dentists, for example, are pretty much "tied to their chairs." They have to make an effort to see other colleagues or join a business association to keep up on the local scuttlebutt. The talk of the day is more than "idle gossip." Knowledge is power and many bits of the information making the rounds can be important to the local practitioner.

Time. In private practice you are always on call. Dentists may be called for painful toothaches at any hour of the day; the obstetrician can always expect a 4:00 a.m. phone call; the surgeon may lose $5–$10,000 by being unavailable on a holiday weekend. One traumatic surgeon who skippered a racing sailboat was reluctant to go racing on a summer weekend, Labor Day, or Memorial Day. Automobile accidents were a major source of his income and he did not feel sufficiently secure financially to be away over a weekend that would probably produce one or two serious accidents.

Stress. The private practitioner takes on the stress of running a business as well as that of patient care. The health professional shares with the businessman the task of meeting a payroll, paying rent, and all the other business commitments associated with staying in business and making a profit. A mental health practitioner who saw patients at a nearby Naval base ran into trouble getting paid because of a regulation that had never been articulated to him: that psychologists were not allowed to treat more than one member of a family. He routinely spoke to the mothers of the children he was treating and sent separate bills for each. This was picked up finally by a clerk. Not only were all his payments held up for several months but he was told he might have to pay the Navy back for all similar billings for which he had been paid. The situation, needless to say, was a stressful one when payment was not forthcoming from an organization with a triple A credit rating like the Navy. (Stress and how to handle it is discussed in detail in Chapter 10.)

In reality the decision to go into private practice will rest on the personality and the inclination of the individual, except for dentistry which is mostly practiced privately and nursing which is to a great extent practiced in institutions or for nurses registries. Mental health practitioners and physicians have a greater range of opportunities and many choose a mixed practice, combining private practice with work on contract to an institution.

A MIXED PRACTICE

The practice of two radiologists in a rural area consists of the following. Their legal identity is that of a corporation. As a corporation they have a contract with the local hospital to deliver X-ray services to patients of the hospital. Each doctor works about half of the time at the hospital, providing full coverage for the hospital from Monday through Friday. In addition they have two other offices; one as a corporation under contract to a local private emergency room and the other is an office of their own which they maintain. As individuals they have a financial interest in the emergency room. With a practice such as theirs with low fees (their average fee is $12) and high volume (they see 25,000 patients a year), they say the best plan is to diversify.

There are other benefits to their arrangements that are less tangible. They work closely with one another, and trust and respect one another both medically and as business partners. Dr. Malone originally bought into the practice and increased the volume of business along with the team of doctors who established and built up the reputation of the new local hospital. Dr. O'Neill joined the practice as an employee for two years and was invited to buy into the corporation. At present they are looking for another associate to follow the same pattern. The advice offered by these radiologists was to buy into an existing practice (1) because radiology is a practice based on referrals (a newcomer cannot hope to break into long-standing referral patterns in an area) and (2) the expenditure for equipment is such a major expense. At the personal and psychological level it was important for both of them to feel a compatibility with each other and with the management of the hospital with which they are associated. Dr. O'Neill did his training in the area but Dr. Malone came to the area from another part of the country.

There are a number of lessons to be drawn from the story of this successful practice. Each specialty, for example, has its own particular problems and advantages. A young pediatrician, for example, or an obstetrician, especially now that the number of births seems to be increasing slightly, might be able to settle in a community where there are a number of older doctors (none of whom are particularly well-liked by the younger women) and have a thriving practice in a year or two. But a lot of legwork would be necessary before a nurse practitioner might be able to establish a successful independent practice in a new community.

A transition period of working for someone else may be a necessary first step. Before making a commitment to a particular community, a dentist might prefer to work in another dentist's office. A mental health practitioner might find employment at a mental health center before establishing a private practice. He or she might then maintain a connection with the center with a contract to supervise or see a number of patients on a weekly basis. Hanging up a shingle and waiting to be discovered as the most knowledgeable, capable, attractive, young practitioner that ever opened an office, is not recommended. Diversification, as the radiologists suggested, keeping your fingers in a lot of pies, seems to be not only more prudent, but a lot more interesting for the practitioner.

Perhaps the most illuminating of the lessons to be gained from the two radiologists is that of the hustle. In private practice you have to hustle. Patients don't just arrive at your doorstep. Much effort must be expended, not just at the outset, but on a continuing basis to make your practice visible in the community and to make and maintain the contacts that will form a referral pattern resulting in a lively practice.

BASIC CHALLENGES

Once the decision is made to enter private practice, there are a number of basic decisions and challenges that the private practitioner must confront.

1. Financial goals: How much money do you want to make?
2. How to meet your financial goals.
   a. Buy into a group practice or work as a salaried employee for a group with the eventual goal of buying into the group.
   b. Buy the practice of a retiring or deceased practitioner.
   c. Work out a mix of private practice and salaried employment in order to meet financial goals while developing a private practice.
3. Where to locate.
   a. Urban versus suburban or even rural.
   b. What section of the country?
   c. Actual location of the office.
4. Rent or buy.
   a. Second office in the home?
5. Develop a referral network.

These are preliminary decisions that must be made before any concrete steps are taken toward opening an office. Some of these decisions will be yours alone to make, for example, whether you will find a group practice more congenial, would prefer to share an office with just one partner, or would prefer to work alone. For other decisions you will require good business advice, perhaps from colleagues or a mentor, if you are fortunate enough to have one. Some decisions, such as the community you choose as the location for your practice, you will want to make after much discussion with your spouse and family. There are even some problems which may seem troublesome at first that just evaporate as solutions fall into place. The whole process may seem overwhelming and even a little frightening, especially if setting up a practice means a move to a new community. However, no decision is irrevocable. But each move should be built on the last one. In this book we have made an attempt to anticipate some of the questions that arise and suggest some possible solutions.

2

Financial planning

WHAT ARE YOUR FINANCIAL GOALS?

One doesn't often meet a man like Dr. Gibbons any more. He was one of the most respected physicians in his suburban community. He taught at a major institution in New York City. But when he died at the age of 50, he left his widow and four children (one at medical school) without a penny. He didn't even own his own home. The explanation is a simple one. He never sent his patients any bills. Dr. Gibbons, like his father before him, was an extreme example of the altruistic, old-fashioned doctor.

Most health professionals want to make a decent living, even though many have chosen their profession for humanitarian reasons. A disdain for money in combination with a strong urge to help people are not the only factors that compete with the money-making urge. Some people don't want to work so hard that they have neither the time nor the energy for family and leisure activities. Women in the helping professions may prefer a private practice just because it gives them the flexibility to combine home and profession in comfortable proportions. Private practice, of course, allows older professionals to cut down on their working day and yet maintain a comfortable income and a sense of purpose. Two young doctors, a husband and wife, set up a family practice in rural New England with a view to putting their roots down deep into that rocky soil, delivering babies, keeping them healthy, and caring for their parents and grandparents. They will make a comfortable living, but never be rich.

For most professionals there is a trade-off between personal goals and financial and professional ones. Personal goals are seldom remunerative. Professional goals, too, may not pay off in monetary terms. Journal articles, research, or working with the disadvantaged, may be satisfying but do not bring in cash.

What are your financial goals? How much money do you want to make? How much money do you want for retirement? When do you want to retire? Do you want to be able to put your children through college? Income can be

TABLE 2-1
Yearly budget for a single person

Housing (rent or mortgage, taxes, fuel) @ $1,000/month	$12,000
Car payments and insurance @ $350/month	4,200
Food	3,000
Clothing	2,000
Telephone and utilities	1,400
Personal expenses, entertainment, and travel	5,000
Appliances, furnishings, and repairs	1,500
Payments on student loans	1,200
Medical, dental, and insurance	1,200
Car expense	2,000
Charity	500
Miscellaneous	1,000
Total	$35,000

planned. A certain number of patients at a specific fee will yield a particular gross income. Expenses can be predicted and a net income after taxes can be calculated. The first step in setting up a private practice is to set your own financial goals in terms of net income. Setting a realistic financial goal will enable you to plan the particular mix of private versus institutional practice needed while you establish your practice. It will help you, too, to allocate your time between personal and professional activities.

Suppose you decide that $35,000 after taxes is a financial goal to aim at. Table 2–1 represents a yearly budget for a single person.

How much money do you need to earn to realize a net income of $35,000. The answer is probably somewhere in the neighborhood of $100,000. Taxes will take $20,000 and the expense of running an office may come close to $45,000.

Calculating office expenses

Does $45,000 for the expenses involved in running an office look high? Let us look at the hypothetical budget in Table 2–2. Forty-five-thousand-plus dollars does not include rental of equipment, interest, and payment on loans, or the purchase of any new equipment either for clinical purposes or office needs.

What about the other side of a financial statement, the income figures? Suppose we stay with our $100,000 income goal. How many patients at $25 a visit does a practitioner have to see to earn $100,000? Your pocket calculator tells you the answer is 4,000 patient visits. That would be 80 patients a week for a 50-week year or 16 patients a day for a five-day week. If you work an eight-hour day, you will be able to spend a half an hour with each patient who comes for an office visit.

These are hypothetical figures that might be applicable to a pediatrician, an internist, a dentist, or a nurse practitioner. The fee of $25 per visit might be too

TABLE 2-2
Hypothetical budget for office expenses for one year

Rent at $750/month	$ 9,000
Salary for receptionist/secretary at $220/week	11,440
Fringe benefits at one third of salary	3,813
Telephone (including Yellow Pages) at $200/month	2,400
Answering service at $40/month	480
Utilities	1,200
Outside services (service contracts) at $120/month	1,440
Disposables (clinical) at $100/month	1,200
Cleaning service at $20/week	1,040
Car expense	6,000
Malpractice insurance	5,000
Liability and theft insurance	750
Professional services (lawyer, accountant)	1,000
Disposables (office)	1,000
Total	$45,763

high or too low for any particular specialty or area. Another way to figure out how to bring in $100,000 is to work out an hourly or weekly charge for your time. You need to make $2,000 a week. If you work an eight-hour day, the hourly rate comes to $50 per hour. That checks out with the first calculation of $25 for a half-hour office visit. (The problem of attracting 4,000 patients a year to your office is discussed in Chapter 5.)

All in all, the hypothetical goal (in reality a modest one) of earning a gross income of $100,000 seems well within the realm of possibility. In the financial planning for opening an office for private practice, the practitioner needs to set financial goals and work out personal and office budgets.

ACHIEVING THE FINANCIAL GOAL FINANCIALLY

At this point you may be wringing your hands. It is all very well to project a modest income to be derived from an overwhelming number of patients with an ongoing office, but you may ask yourself, "how do I project myself into this picture. I have spent every nickel I could beg and borrow to get myself through school and I owe the government thousands of dollars in student loans." The answer is to borrow more from your friendly neighborhood banker.

Financing and risk

Most people hate to be in debt. "Never a borrower or a lender be" was the advice of old Polonius. Such advice may be fine for personal conduct but it does not apply to business. Borrowing, or financing, the business term, is vital to the business world. In fact, a loan increases your net worth, since a loan is counted as an asset. Borrowing, contrary to oft-stated attitudes, is respectable. One man described it like this. "When I started in business I was broke. Now I owe a million dollars and am one of the leading citizens in my community." Or as one author put it, "If you owe $50, you are a delinquent account. If you owe $50,000, you are a small businessman. If you owe $50 million, you are a corporation. If you owe $50 billion, you are a government." In other words, the more money you owe, the greater respect and influence you command.

A word of caution is necessary. A business borrows money as a tool to make money. And therein lies the source of respect. As a health practitioner/business-person, you will borrow money to set up your business and for use as working capital. *Do not borrow money for living expenses.* You cannot realize any profit when you are living on borrowed money.

The disadvantage of borrowing lies in the risk you are taking. You have to pay back the money plus the interest on the loan, the cost of borrowing. That means you must make a leap of faith, that is, take the risk that you will be able to do so by the practice of your profession. But you may not be able to attract patients. You may get sick. You may mismanage the business aspects of the practice. These are the risks that every businessperson takes—that things will go wrong or that you have miscalculated.

Planning

There are ways to minimize the risk. Essentially this involves planning. There are a number of questions to be answered—the very questions that a banker will ask before granting a loan. First, how much money do you need and what do you plan to do with it? Second, how do you plan to pay back the loan? A third question for you to think about concerns the kind of money you want to borrow—that is, the length of time you need the money and the source of funds for repayment of the loan. Both are related to the purpose for which the funds are to be used.

Short-term loans. You can use short-term money for such purposes as financing accounts receivable for 30 or 60 days or as long as six months. Usually lenders expect short-term loans to be paid back when the purpose has been achieved as, for example, when patients have paid their bills.

There are sources other than commercial banks for short-term loans. The Household Finance Corporation may have less stringent requirements for a loan, although their interest rates may be higher than the commercial banks. MasterCharge and Visa are a source of short-term money. You will probably want to establish a line of credit with these credit companies as well as with your own bank in case of a sudden need for business funds. An overdraft on your checking account is also a source for short-term funds. "Think before you leap" is the motto for tapping this readily accessible money. These should be considered sources of last resort in cases of extreme need. A short-term loan must be paid back quickly because the cost of borrowing is high.

Long-term loans. The purpose of a long-term loan might be to set up your office or to buy an expensive piece of equipment. The best way to think about a long-term loan is as money you will pay back in periodic installments over a fairly long period of time, such as from three to seven years.

The unsecured loan. This is the most frequently used form of bank credit for short-term purposes. You do not have to put up collateral because the bank relies on your credit reputation or, in other words, your record as a borrower in paying back a loan.

The secured and/or cosigned loan. A pledge of some or all of your heretofore unsecured assets is required. There are other kinds of collateral. Borrowers sometimes have other people cosign a note with them in order to bolster their own credit. However, the endorser or cosigner becomes liable for the note if you, the borrower, fail to pay up. Sometimes the endorser is asked to put up assets also. Or you might get a loan by putting up a savings account from another bank. Banks may also accept the unencumbered cash value of a life insurance policy as collateral. Stocks and bonds are another form of collateral, but you will probably not get more than 75 percent of the value of high grade securities or up to 90 percent of the market value of federal or municipal bonds.

Equity capital. This is the kind of money that you don't have to pay back. You offer a part ownership in your business to a person or people who are willing to take a risk. They are interested in potential income rather than an immediate return on their investment.

HOW MUCH DO YOU NEED TO BORROW?

Let us say you want to open an office for the first time and you are planning to borrow money from the bank to help you get started. You will need several months rent, office furniture and equipment, clinical supplies, and office supplies. You plan to paint and redecorate. With the help of an accountant, draw up a budget to see how much it will cost just to open your doors. Table 2–3 suggests some of the items you will have to consider.

TABLE 2–3
Budget of expenses to open office

Phone equipment and installation	$ 500
Examining room equipment and supplies	2,500
Office equipment and supplies	2,500
Advertising (Yellow Pages, newspaper announcements)	500
Printing (stationery, announcements)	750
Checks, bookkeeping supplies, bills (one-write system)	500
Decorating office (paint, linoleum, carpeting)	1,500
Professional services (lawyer)	750
Miscellaneous	500
Total	$10,000

Large capital expenses, such as dental operatorium, may cost $35,000 over seven years plus debt service.

Our hypothetical figures show a capital budget of $10,000. This money can be borrowed on a long-term loan. Let's say you will pay it back over a five-year period. Suppose you decide to ask for a $7,500 long-term loan. The interest and pay-back schedule will run roughly at $200 a month which you will have to take account of in your operating budget.

Operating budget

Your operating budget will show recurring monthly expenses whereas the capital expenses occur only once. Some suggested figures are shown in Table 2–4.

TABLE 2-4
Operating expenses per month

Rent	$ 500
Salary for secretary/receptionist	1,000
Utilities	100
Phone	100
Answering service	40
Linen service	30
Cleaning services	80
Postage	20
Disposables (office and clinical)	100
Interest and amortization on long-term loan	200
Total	$2,170

Cash budget

You will spend more than you earn for awhile until the payment of fees starts to catch up with expenditures. You cannot really begin to figure out how much money to borrow for operating expense or how you are going to repay a short-term loan for that purpose until you know at what point in time your income will begin to catch up with operating expenses.

When you have worked out a projected budget for monthly expenses, the next step is to work out a projected monthly cash income. Table 2-5 is based on

TABLE 2-5
Estimated monthly income from new practice from January to June

	January	February	March	April	May	June
Number of patients	20	40	60	80	100	120
January	$250	$250				
February		$500	$ 500			
March			$ 750	$ 750		
April				$1,000	$1,000	
May					$1,250	$1,250
June						$1,500
Monthly income	$250	$750	$1,250	$1,750	$2,250	$2,750

a starting patient load of 20 people per month, increasing at the rate of 20 patients per month, with 120 patient/visits in the month of June. For purposes of illustration we will assume a fee of $25 per visit and that half the patients pay in the month they are seen and the remaining half pay the following month.

Now you are ready to calculate an estimate of your borrowing requirements by means of a cash budget. You will notice that the estimated monthly expense budget does not include a salary for the practitioner. Let us make the assumption that the practitioner will work at a clinic four mornings a week at $25 per hour for a weekly income of $400. This will pay personal and automobile expenses. Also it is recommended that you try to keep a $500 balance in the checking account. A cash budget for six months based on the hypothetical expenses and income projected in the above charts is calculated in Table 2-6.

TABLE 2-6
Cash budget showing an estimate of borrowing requirements

	January	Febuary	March	April	May	June	July
Cash requirements:							
Operating expenses	$2,160	$2,160	$2,160	$2,160	$2,160	$2,160	$2,160
Cash available:							
Collections	250	750	1,250	1,750	2,250	2,750	3,250
Excess cash over receipts	0	0	0	0	90	590	1,090
Additional cash required	1,910	1,410	910	410	0	0	0

A total of the additional cash requirements for the months of January through May equals $4,640. Rounding off this figure to $5,000 will provide close to $500 for the checking account in the month of April to take care of any bills that may come due at that time. These figures show that repayment on the loan can begin by the end of June and can reach the rate of $1,000 a month by July if the practice continues to expand. At $1,000 a month the loan can be repaid by the end of November. Five thousand dollars would probably be made available as an unsecured loan in the form of a line of credit to be used as necessary.

The larger sum you need is the $7,500 for capital expenses. Before looking for a cosigner among your relatives and friends, you might try to borrow the money on the basis of your own *net worth*. You may be able to convince a banker that you are an excellent credit risk—an able health professional, a personable and responsible individual who will attract patients and keep them, with a respectable net worth.

Personal finances

A statement of net worth includes every asset and liability you have that can in any way be represented by a monetary sum. Remember to list property that may seem of dubious value such as the old saxophone you lent to your nephew and your microscope from medical school. Figure 2-1 shows a form that will

FIGURE 2-1

FINANCIAL STATEMENT

Assets		Liabilities	
Cash and checking	_____	Mortgages	_____
Savings accounts	_____	Notes payable	_____
Real estate owned	_____	Loans on life insurance	_____
Securities	_____	Debts, unsecured	_____
Notes receivable	_____	Installment purchases	_____
Bonds—face value	_____	Property tax reserves	_____
Furniture and personal	_____	Income tax reserves	_____
Automobiles	_____	Judgments against you	_____
Life insurance cash value	_____		
Boats and trailers	_____		
Alimony	_____		
Other	_____		
	_____		
	_____		
Total assets	_____	Total liabilities	_____

Net worth _____

help you. You may be surprised at your net worth after you have added up the figures.

SEEKING A BANK LOAN

It is important to remember that banks are in the business of making loans. They accept deposits from their depositors and make a profit by lending that money out. That is to say, when you go to a banker you are not asking for charity. On the other hand, the banker has an obligation to the bank's depositors not to lose their money. That gives bankers the right to ask a lot of questions. When you go to a bank to ask to borrow money, you are in effect making the bank a silent partner in your business. Their right to ask pertinent questions about your business, your financial worth, and your character is based on their need to assess the likelihood that you will be able to keep to your side of the contract and pay back the loan according to the agreed upon terms.

In addition, some bankers can provide valuable financial counsel and criticism. They may have an intimate knowledge of the financial affairs of many businesses and may have lent money to the health professionals in the community. The closer the relationship between the professional and the banker, the more effective the banker can be in helping to finance the professional's practice.

In granting an unsecured loan, the bank's loan committee usually relies on a favorable evaluation of the borrower's four "C's"—character, condition, capital, and credit. And the most important of these is character. Character includes the bank's estimate of how well you handle money as well as your personal honesty. Condition in business refers to the firm, the industry, and the product. For the health professional, the bank would be interested in your professional ability as well as the competitiveness of your specialty in the community. If you are a dentist and the bank happens to know that three of the eight dentists in town are having trouble making ends meet, they may discourage you from opening an office in the area. Capital refers to the individual's investment in the practice and the bank's assessment of the ability of the borrower to pay back the loan. Credit refers to the reputation and history of the professional for repayment of loans—a good reason for taking seriously the obligation to repay student loans.

If you have never asked for a business loan before, it might be helpful for you to make an appointment with a loan officer and ask for some suggestions about the lending process: What documents to bring, what kinds of terms are likely to be offered, what questions to be prepared to answer. In addition to projected budgets, income estimates, and a cash-flow projection (cash budget), you might be asked for copies of your federal income tax returns for the last few years. You will probably be asked about the insurance you carry. Take the loan application home with you and study it. You might want to consult with your accountant and/or your lawyer.

Negotiating with the bank

Ask to see the papers you will need to sign before you close on the loan. You may not like the terms that are being offered. The bank may have put certain limitations on the loan such as the repayment terms, the pledging or the use of security, and periodic reporting. The actual restrictions come under the heading of covenants which may be negative or positive. Negative covenants forbid a borrower from certain actions such as making further additions to the borrower's total debt and pledging to others the borrower's assets. Positive covenants spell out things that the borrower must do, such as maintaining a minimum of net working capital, carrying of adequate insurance, and supplying the lender with financial statements from time to time.

You can negotiate. If you don't like the terms, say so. If the bank thinks you are a good credit risk, and health professionals are most often considered good loan prospects, they may make a more favorable offer. You may want to consult with colleagues or other advisors. In short, try to get terms you can live with. Remember that once the terms have been agreed upon, there is little that can be done to change them afterwards.

3

Establishing an office

CHOOSING A LOCATION

Let us assume that you have decided to open up your own practice and you can manage the financing for such a step. Where should you establish yourself? Some people know from the outset, or decide early on, that they will practice in their own home town. This may be an excellent choice if there is a referral network open to them and they can count on access to one or more of the local hospitals. Although some women may encounter more prejudice against them as physicians among colleagues and patients who knew them as little girls, the female nurse practitioner may find old friendships and associations an excellent foundation on which to build a successful practice. Physicians may decide to practice in the city where they finished training. This offers the advantage of knowing most of the doctors in their own specialty as well as many other doctors who might be possible sources of referral. However, since many others make the same choice, they may find their services are not in great demand.

Because a health practice is a portable profession, provided that state requirements are fulfilled, you may be among those who are looking over several broad regions for just the right area and community in which to practice and make a home. This will be an important choice. What are some of the factors you should consider? First and foremost will be the need in the community for your specialty. Then, you will want to check on the general economic conditions of the area. Is the economy expanding? What kind of people live there? Are they rich or poor? Old or young? In the final analysis, those professional factors may not be as important to your overall satisfaction with the area and the community, as the many personal reasons which direct your choice. Will the place be one in which you and your spouse want to live? There are, then, three major considerations in choosing a location: personal, financial, and professional.

What kind of a place do you want to live in?

Frequently when professionals move to a new area they do so for personal rather than business reasons. You are invited for a visit out of state and you get the feeling in your bones that the area would be a good one for you. You like the look of it. The gas station attendant is helpful. The people you meet at a party seem genuinely eager to have you move to the community. Many people are almost embarrassed to explain why they located in a particular area. Do you sail, ski, or fish? Will the dry air alleviate your allergies? Do you hate winter? Do you have a good friend or family members in an area? These are all perfectly adequate reasons to consider locating in a community.

But lest first impressions prove insubstantial, you had better make a more thorough investigation of the community to see if it is really a place where you and your family want to live.

Will you be able to find a suitable home reasonably close to the hospital and a possible office site?

If you have children, you will want to find out if the schools are doing a good job with their students.

Read the local paper, watch the local TV station, and listen to the local radio station. Is this a community in which there are a fair number of people who share your political, religious, and philosophical outlook?

Will you encounter problems due to your ethnic, racial, or religious background?

If you are a joiner and enjoy committee work, are there community organizations you will be able to support and participate in?

What about recreational activities for you and your family? Little League? a community orchestra? indoor tennis?

The economics and demographics of the area

Your personal success will be determined not only by your competence and personal characteristics, but also by the particular economic and demographic conditions in the area. Statistics compiled by the Bureau of the Census and other government agencies can take much of the guesswork out of the nature of the economic climate of an area that seems promising for opening a private practice. The Bureau of the Census breaks the country down into Standard Metropolitan Statistical Areas (SMSAs). An SMSA contains a central city of at least 50,000, plus neighboring areas that are economically and socially integrated into the central city. An SMSA is divided into smaller statistical units called census tracts. The average census tract has about 4,000–5,000 inhabitants. In urban areas there are even smaller geographical units—block statistics—within a census tract. By comparing different census tracts in an area you may be able to choose a location for your office with a growing population, a high per capita income, a well-educated population. Information from the Bureau of the Census tract about a particular SMSA and census is often available at local libraries or the publications may be used or purchased at the United States Department of Commerce district offices, located in 43 major cities.

Population. The Bureau of the Census counts not only the number of people in a given area, but their age, and the gain or loss of people. Are most of your patients children or adolescents? Are there a good proportion of young people in the child-bearing ages? Do you see mostly older people? Florida, for example, has more older people than any other state.

Wealth. The socioeconomic characteristics of an area can be revealed by a number of indicators: unemployment, labor force characteristics, i.e., the kind of work performed by people who are working, the level of education, i.e., years of school completed, and family income. Occupation, education, and income statistics are strongly related. People with a higher level of education will tend to have higher level jobs and a higher income. Is a state gaining or losing population? The 1980 census showed that Rhode Island and New York were losing population, whereas Nevada, New Mexico and Florida (among others) were gaining. A comparison of several census tracts in an area may be necessary since inflation introduces a distortion into income figures.

Unemployment. What is the rate of unemployment? A number of states in the middle west—North and South Dakota, Nebraska, and Kansas, for example, have the lowest rates. On the other hand, North and South Dakota are among the poorer states in respect to per capita income. Kansas, however, is a fairly rich state.

Economic growth. Another factor important to the health practitioner is economic growth. What are the business trends in a state? Are they losing or gaining in the number of businesses? Is the local economy dependent on one industry or even one company? If so, what is the economic health of the industry or company? Driving around a community can reveal economic realities. Is there any building activity? Are the public buildings, parks, schools, and other facilities well maintained? Are the stores busy? Is there a good selection of fresh produce, meat, and other groceries in the local supermarket?

A few words of caution are in order. Each set of statistics requires interpretation. One dentist did some research, found a high density of population and a low ratio of dentists per capita only to find an inordinately high unemployment rate and a population that would be more inclined to go to a clinic than a dentist in private practice (Gehrman, 1981). Ideally, for a financially successful practice you would want to choose an area with a growing population, especially in the age groups that form your patient pool, a well-educated and comparatively wealthy population, and a rising number of businesses moving in.

It must be remembered that conditions are not uniform in a state. Even in a state that is losing population, like Rhode Island, and that is sparsely settled outside of the one major population area, there are areas of business and population growth as well as economically active enclaves that offer an opportunity for a health practitioner.

Competition

Having satisfied yourself that the community you have chosen can be justified on a sound economic and business basis, there are a number of factors that will have a bearing on the success of your private practice. The most important of these is the need for your specialty and the competition from others who have already established their practices.

An area will support only a certain number of practitioners in any particular field. Moving into an already saturated area can be difficult. Referral patterns are difficult to break into, hospital staff membership may be closed, and civic groups well supplied with speakers. Particularly crucial is the number of practitioners in your specialty. How many plastic surgeons specializing in cosmetic surgery can a community support?

You may find that a community you have found congenial to live in, that is also in a healthy economic condition, has attracted others in your field. One psychotherapist opened an office in a small university town with a growing population, located halfway between two hospitals, and in which there were no other mental health practitioners. Much to his dismay two other psychotherapists opened offices in town the same year.

There is no way to anticipate or avoid such unknown competition, but an afternoon in the library of the local hospital will provide information on the competition in your specialty in a given community. The American Medical Association and the American Dental Association have published information on the distribution of practitioners by state, region, district, and county. Use the *Directory of Medical Specialists* to make a list of the specialists in your field in your chosen community. *The National Register of Health Service Providers in Psychology* and *The National Register of Certified Social Workers* will show the distribution of practitioners in these fields. However, a healthy ratio of physicians per capita or a desirable ratio of specialists to other physicians in an area varies so according to economic and demographic conditions that no hard and fast rules can be made. There is no substitute for a trip to the area to call on the local health professionals.

Ask the local practitioners. The directories will provide the addresses and names of the directors of the state and county medical associations as well as the hospital administrators. Dentists and nurse practitioners can obtain this information from their own professional organizations. Make a list also of the primary care physicians or local dentists, nurses, mental health practitioners, as the case may be. Plan your trip in advance. Make appointments ahead with the organizational directors, hospital administrators, specialists in your field, and even primary care physicians, dentists, and nurses. Many people welcome the chance to display their knowledge of their community, gossip about their colleagues, and talk business to a potential newcomer. As always, a thank-you note will not go unnoticed by a future colleague and referral source.

The executive director of the local medical (dental, nurse's) association will perhaps be the single best informant on your list. Despite his or her professional discretion, you will be able to get a sense from what is said as well as what is not said, of the local medical scene. He (she) knows many of the local health practitioners and may be willing to suggest which ones would be most profitable for you to see. Hospital administrators are also a good source for information on the need for your specialty and your prospective competition.

The specialists in your field are, finally, the best judges of the need of another practitioner. Do they have more patients than they can comfortably handle? Or are they finding their waiting rooms empty?

Restrictions. Fear of competition may bring about restrictions for the new-comer. State licensing arrangements may place barriers in the way of older practitioners who are planning a move to a warmer climate. One successful dentist took the South Carolina boards because he wanted to move to Hilton Head Island. He failed the practicals. If you are thinking of such an eventual move, it might be well to take boards now in Florida, California, Arizona, and other of the sunbelt states and to keep that license active (Gehrman, 1981).

Choose an important medical center. An exception to avoiding competition would be to open a practice in an area famous for excellent health facilities. Health practitioners as well as patients tend to gravitate to areas with one or more major hospitals and specialists in many fields. For a physician with a subspecialty—a pediatrician, for example, in adolescent medicine—the presence of other pediatricians may be advantageous. They will in fact be a source of referrals as their patients reach the teen years. Such an area would be an excellent place for a nurse practitioner who would be able to guide patients in the management of their medical difficulties. In addition, if an area is known for its health facilities, there may be a halo effect, that is, patients may consider a doctor to be better qualified to treat them if they practice in that area.

URBAN, SUBURBAN, RURAL

Health practitioners, like most people who have the choice, prefer for the most part to live outside of large cities. The older cities of the Northeast, the Middle West and the South are contending with a myriad of problems—fiscal, economic, and social. Crime, deterioration of the basic public services, poverty, and racial conflict are the daily facts of urban life. To live well in a large city is costly. Rents are high; ownership is even more expensive; and you may want to send your children to private school. On the other hand, country life and a country practice has an appeal to only a few. To make the choice involves a whole spectrum of personal preferences from those of lifestyle to professional and financial goals.

Are you a city person?

There is no doubt that the most important medical centers are still located in the large urban centers. Medical practitioners who want to be at the cutting edge of their profession will want to practice and be affiliated with a major teaching hospital. You can keep up with the latest developments and get to know the key people in your field. And it may be easier to become affiliated with a hospital in a large city than in the suburbs or a small city where the department chiefs may have a stranglehold on appointments. If your training was in a large city hospital, you will already have the advantage of professional and personal relationships and will be in a better position to make a place for yourself.

Your professional specialty may dictate your decision. Large medical centers attract patients from a wide radius to be treated by physicians with narrowly defined areas of specialization. The orthopedist who specializes in microsurgery for knee injuries will need to locate near a major medical facility. Patients will come many miles for treatment. Oral surgeons who do only complex maxillofacial procedures will look for a location near a central city. Rents and salaries are higher than the suburbs, but the trade-off is higher fees. The equipment owned by a major hospital, too, may determine the specialists' location. Is a CAT scan available for the neurologist or a team trained in heart transplant procedures, for the heart specialist? The specialties practised at the medical facility itself will determine the location of a practice for many specialists.

Large cities also tend to divide into neighborhoods centered around schools, churches, and areas for shopping. An urban residential neighborhood will support an array of health practitioners such as dentists, internists, family practitioners, and pediatricians. Specialists in preventive medicine, mental health, and health education such as the nurse practitioners, the group therapist, the sex therapist may find many patients among the sophisticated population of an urban neighborhood.

Finally, however, the decision to locate in an urban area is a matter of personal preference. If your family lives in the suburbs while you practice in the city, it is you who will face the daily commutation and time spent away from your family. If you are a city person, you will accept the discomforts of city life and see instead the advantages of a more cosmopolitan frame of reference, of being able to live a private life completely separate from your profession, of sharing in the excitement of the urban milieu.

A suburban practice

In the last 25 or 30 years, health practitioners have joined the escape from the city to the suburbs. First-rate hospitals are now well established in most suburbs. Where there may have been a few general practitioners, dentists, and obstetricians 25 years ago, now all but the most arcane specialists abound. This generation of middle-class mothers would not consider going to the city to have their babies, whereas their mothers may have traveled 20 miles or more to a major city where they were born. Although some suburbs may now have become oversaturated in many specialties, that first generation of health practitioners who followed their patients to the suburbs may now be getting ready to retire. The children of the baby boom of the late 1940s are now returning to the suburbs to bring up their own children. As the population turns over, there is once again a need for young health practitioners.

For graduating medical students looking ahead, an internship and residency in the town or suburb where they eventually want to practice is an excellent idea. Or conversely, to make the decision to stay where they train has many advantages. Principal among them are the contacts and relationships made with the established practitioners in town. These people will form the basis for a referral pattern in the future. In addition, many relationships are set up with patients who constitute the basis for a patient referral pattern.

Despite the obvious advantages of living in a suburb or a small city, there is the possible disadvantage that the health practitioner, like the religious leader, is always on view. There is not the anonymity of an urban area. Judgments are made. There may be expectations by the community that health practitioners will participate in community affairs, give generously to local charities, and be models for the next generation. Neighbors may note how you bring up your children and judge them as well. This may or may not be your cup of tea. You may enjoy being seen around town and recognized by one and all. Or you may attempt to keep a low profile.

A country practice

In rural areas everyone knows everybody's business. Also, if you are the only medical practitioner in the immediate area, you will be expected to care for all emergencies and will essentially always be on call. But rural places offer a unique compensation to some—that of living in the country and knowing its inhabitants well. For the nurse practitioner and the family practitioner, there is a good living—better than that of most country people and expenses are low. A small town is not a place to make a lot of money; rather, its rewards are the quiet kind—putting down roots and experiencing the relationship of people and the natural world.

As noted in the Preface, medical economics are changing in rural areas due to a greater supply of physicians graduating from medical school than of doctors who are retiring or dying. Many small communities, no longer suffering from a shortage of doctors, have become centers for medical care for the surrounding countryside. New hospitals attract specialists. If a sufficient proportion of the population in the area carries medical insurance, financial support for private practitioners becomes a reality. So for health professionals who are attracted to the rural life, care in choosing a small town can now result in not only the capability of practicing modern medicine in a well-equipped hospital with competent colleagues, but the assurance of a perfectly adequate standard of living.

CHOOSING AN OFFICE SITE

The ideal site for a health practitioner differs from the small retail business in that the health practitioner does not have to attract people off the street. A person may pass by a health practitioner's office four times daily and it would never occur to her to walk in, except possibly in an emergency. On the other hand, the address should not be obscure. The office should be centrally located and easy to find. The directions for getting there should be easy to explain over the phone. Probably the street name should not be too difficult to spell or to pronounce. It should be accessible to public transportation. And there should be adequate parking space. Most important, it should be convenient for you—not too far from your home, not too far from your hospital, and not too far from your clinic or other locations where you keep regular hours. A good rule of thumb might be that not more than 10 minutes should be spent driving from any one of those places to any other.

Locating near a hospital

Generally there is office space available for medical practitioners near a hospital—professional offices designed for medical practice. These may consist of a series of residences converted to offices (doctor's row) or one or more office buildings designed specifically for health professionals.

There are a number of advantages to an office across the street from the hospital, especially for those who must be at the hospital once or more each day. Obstetricians can see patients in their office and be on call, knowing that they can reach the delivery room in just a few moments. A doctor whose practice involves a good deal of hospital consultation will lose no time in travel to the hospital. Frequent association and contact with other doctors in the building or on the street offer the advantage of becoming part of a referral network. And finally, such locations are usually prestigious. The important specialists are frequently located in office space near a hospital. To have your office among them puts you in their company.

The major disadvantage is the cost. However, you may be able to offset some of the higher rental by sharing such expenses as receptionist, waiting room, and secretarial and billing services with a colleague.

Some doctors maintain an office in a hospital. Hospital arrangements vary. In addition to supplying space, a hospital may provide clerical and receptionist services, telephone, and, most important, equipment. The doctor, in turn, may have to observe certain hours. With your office in the hospital, you will have the advantage of referrals, not only from the other doctors, but from the hospital emergency room.

Should you practice in your own home?

Maintaining your principal (or even an auxiliary) office in your own home has certain tax advantages. You can deduct a percentage of the cost of operating and maintaining your house according to the ratio of office space to total space in the house. If, for example, you use two of the eight rooms in your house for an office, you may deduct 25 percent of such expenses as heat, electricity, mortgage payments, repairs, painting, cleaning service, snow removal, and other expenses incurred as a part of home ownership.

In addition to the tax advantages, there is a saving in the time and cost of transportation. One's home is most convenient in an emergency. For those with children or other domestic responsibilities, an office in the home offers the unique advantage of maintaining a practice without leaving the house. One can supervise household activities and be available when children are ill. There may be other personal reasons for a practice in the home.

Practitioners who choose to practice at home should arrange their office to be completely separate from the rest of the house. Intimate and homely incidents, no matter how charming, can destroy the respect and confidence a patient may have in the professional expertise of a health practitioner. One's personal life should be invisible.

Zoning restrictions. If you decide to buy a house which will serve you both as a home and an office, check the local zoning regulations. Most communities restrict the uses to which particular areas may be put. Zoning regulations designate certain areas and even specific streets for residential, commercial, or manufacturing use. In most communities health practitioners and other professionals are permitted to locate their offices in their homes, but frequently there are restrictions on the size of the staff. Such regulations protect a residentially zoned area from undue traffic, excessive parking, and other undesirable disturbances.

It is often possible to obtain a variance from the zoning board if your plans for a home office do not meet local requirements. Such a procedure usually entails the sending of letters to neighbors within a certain distance of the property to invite them to a hearing at which the zoning board hears the merits of the case and makes a ruling. Your contract to buy a particular house should be contingent upon your being able to use a portion of the house for an office and to obtain a variance from the zoning board if it is necessary. If there has been prior and continued use of a property as a doctor's or dentist's office in an area restricting such use, with no interruption in occupancy, then the location may continue to be used for such purposes. A doctor with a busy practice may have had an office in a restricted area before the zoning regulations were made, which would account for such an exception.

LEASE OR BUILD

Owning your own office may be one of the best investments a health practitioner can make. Health practitioners are their own best tenants. They can rest assured the rent will be paid. They have their own best interests in keeping up the building and the surrounding area. And they can build and divide to suit themselves. For the dentist or physician with special requirements, such as a multiple practice with many small rooms and a consequent patient-flow problem or special equipment requirements, building to suit may constitute the best solution. You can set up a corporation to own the building (of which you are the principal stockholder) and rent the space to yourself.

On the other hand, there are a number of drawbacks to owning and building an office early in your practice. Principal among them is the time and effort spent in planning and supervising the construction as well as the business aspects of developing the property. Too much brain power and too much capital can be tied up in a building that is peripheral to a health practice. Most health professionals who eventually build their own office or alter an existing building for that purpose, do so after they have established a successful practice.

Leasing

A lease is a legal contract with a landlord that stipulates the conditions under which you occupy the space he or she owns, including the rent you pay. Have your lawyer read the lease. A good lawyer can alert you to omissions or stipulations you may regret not having been aware of.

Do not take anything for granted. Inspect the premises for defects. Turn the faucets on and off. Do the doors and windows open and shut properly? Can they be locked and are the premises sufficiently burglar-proof to satisfy your insurance company? Do you need more electrical outlets? Are there any funny noises when the people next door flush a toilet or use any machinery? It may be well worth the small investment to hire a contractor, inspector, or appraiser to make a complete inspection of the premises including the wiring, plumbing, parking lot, hardware and locks, alarm system, if any, and any mechanical appliances such as a hot water heater.

Improvements to the premises should be specified as a part of the lease. If possible be sure that repairs, painting, and other work is done before your lease starts. Do not assume the work has been done. Make your own inspection before you sign the lease. Even if the promise is made that everything will be done—"not to worry"—it will be time consuming and annoying to have to hound the landlord to keep those promises after you have moved in.

Several other stipulations should be considered. Does the landlord pay all maintenance costs? If you are subleasing from another tenant and are sharing costs, do you share waiting room space? Does the rent include the receptionist and the cleaning costs? If you are planning to take a larger space than you can presently use, is there any objection to your renting out space to other professionals? Are the premises open on Sundays and holidays? Are the parking lot, entrance, and hallways lit in the evening, if you plan to keep evening office hours?

A lease with a future. If you are just starting out in practice, how long a commitment should you make? Under the present uncertain economic conditions a long-term lease may prove impractical. A short-term lease that runs for a year or 18 months will give you sufficient time to test a specific geographic location without imposing too great a financial obligation. Since most leases are now tied to the cost-of-living index or the cost of fuel, there may be little advantage to a longer lease. However, if the landlord does extensive renovation to accommodate your requirements, a longer lease may be expected.

A lease with an option to buy. If you are planning an extensive alteration of the premises and the location is good, you might want to consider a lease with an option to buy. Such a lease will stipulate a price for the property. Short of an option to buy, you might negotiate for the right of first refusal, an arrangement whereby the landlord must offer the property to you before selling it to anyone else. To establish a price, the owner finds another purchaser who agrees to buy the property at a specific price. That price is the one you will have to meet, if you decide to pick up your right of first refusal.

Gross lease and net lease. In addition to being tied to an escalator clause such as the price of fuel or the cost-of-living, a lease can stipulate that all you are buying is the right to occupy the premises. You must pay all other costs, including maintenance, heat, taxes, and utilities. This is known as a gross lease. A net lease would require the owner to pay such costs. A lease may also stipulate that you pay any combination of such costs. Some gross leases are cheaper, as the tenant assumes nearly all aspects of maintenance and management of the property. On the other hand, the trouble and the bookkeeping will be passed on to you. However, since management of property is a business in its own right, it scarcely seems sensible for a health practitioner to spend time and effort managing the rental property he or she occupies.

HOW MUCH SPACE CAN YOU AFFORD?

The cost of commercial space is reckoned by the square foot per year—although you may be quoted a monthly rental for a particular office space. Thus a 500-square-foot space at $7 a square foot will have an annual rental of $3,500 or roughly $300 a month.

Rental costs vary according to location, the condition of the building, and the services provided. For raw space, that is, space that has not been altered to accommodate a medical or dental practice, you may pay anywhere from $6 to $12 a square foot in a small city or a suburb. In the downtown area of a sizable city, rentals may run from $15 to $20 a square foot. Rentals in major cities in a fashionable location are considerably more.

How many square feet you will need depends, of course, on your practice. But a number of generalizations can be made. The following are minimum areas:

Psychotherapist. The psychotherapist will probably have the smallest and simplest office of any health practitioner. The psychotherapist beginning a practice might need 350 square feet, but be able to make do with 150 square feet—a consultation room and a small waiting room, ideally with an exit door from the consultation room.

Waiting room—75 square feet. Room enough for a couple of chairs and an end table.

Consultation room—100 square feet. The size of a small bedroom. This will allow for a desk, several soft chairs and a couch, and even a filing cabinet. It will accommodate three or four people.

Group therapy—200 square feet. To accommodate eight people sitting in chairs.

Secretary's area—less than 100 square feet. Probably not needed for the beginning psychotherapist. A desk, typewriter, and supplies might be built into a closet.

Physician. The physician at the start of his or her practice will need more space than indicated above. For a physician beginning a practice, 500 square feet might be a size to use for comparison when shopping for office space.

Waiting room—Minimum of 40 square feet plus 10 square feet per individual using the room.

Secretary's area—The secretary's area is often placed adjacent to the waiting room, set apart by a low partition. A combination waiting room/secretary's area might require 150 to 200 square feet, room for filing cabinets, supplies, secretarial desk and chair, and five or six waiting patients.

Examining rooms—80 square feet. An area 8' x 10' is sufficient. A physician beginning a practice might require two examining rooms.

Consultation room—100 square feet for a desk and chair and several chairs for patient and companion.

Sharing the cost. A strategy for lowering overhead costs, especially in the initial stages of a practice, might be for two or more practitioners to share space in which to see private patients. Mental health practitioners who divide their practice between private patients and institutional commitments, might work out an arrangement with one or two colleagues to use an office at different hours or share a larger room for group therapy sessions. Nurse practitioners, too, often find it economical to share space. Physicians sometimes share space as well as a receptionist and a nurse, but do not necessarily practice as partners. Care must be taken, just as in a partnership, to spell out the procedure that will be followed if one of the colleagues decides to move out before the lease is up.

4

Recruiting and supervising staff

RECRUITING STAFF

Even if you begin your practice in the most humble fashion—answering your own phone, sending out your own bills, keeping your own books, and perhaps having a public stenographer type your letters, you will soon be too busy to be both practitioner and office manager. You will need people, if at first only on a part-time basis, to take over the administrative aspects of your practice. It is scarcely cost efficient for you to be doing work that can be performed by a nonprofessional at a comparatively low cost.

Administrative staff must be recruited, trained, and supervised. Since you will be paying the salary—be the boss—the burden falls on you. If your staff is a large one, you will not be directly involved with supervising each employee. Nevertheless the atmosphere of the office, whether it be friendly, businesslike, abrupt, or downright nasty, is your responsibility. What kind of people do you want to surround yourself with? How do you get them to do what you want? And how do you see to it that they are doing their job?

The first person a prospective patient talks to is the person who answers your phone. When that patient arrives at the door, he or she will not be greeted by you but by a member of your staff. The impression, we might say the "vibes," the patient picks up from your staff conveys the tone of your practice and even of your personality. Are you easy going? Or all business? Are you compulsive about keeping to your appointment book, or do you have time for a personal consideration of each patient? Of course, you don't want to, and, in fact, would not be able to, hire people who have your personality characteristics. However, you do want people who understand the ambience that you are trying to create and will lend themselves to it. You would scarcely want to hire someone who hated kids, if you are a pedodontist, or someone who had no patience for old people if you are an internist.

Other qualities to look for in a potential employee, for example, a receptionist/secretary, are the elementary ones of punctuality, neat appearance, and reliability. Beyond that you would want to hire a person who speaks well with a good telephone voice and personality, a person who is intelligent, and who listens. If you are looking for a part-time worker, you will need a person whose schedule will fit yours and for whom there is no transportation problem.

Job descriptions

In addition to a candidate's personal characteristics, you will want to hire a person who will be able to perform certain specific duties. What is it exactly that you want an office assistant to do? The best way to define these duties is to write a job description. This may seem like so much bureaucratic red tape, but it is a useful exercise. It will fix in your mind what you expect an assistant to do. It also will define for the employee the substance as well as the limits of the job. Most important to an employee, a job description puts an employer on notice that an employee cannot be expected to do everything. As you write a job description, remember that it is a tool and subject to change and modification. A job description also forms an important part of the interview with a prospective employee. After an initial interview you might want to add to these duties or negotiate some changes. A sample job description for an office assistant might read as follows:

> Answer the phone, keep the appointment book, make appointments, and handle billing, patient accounts, and insurance forms. Take dictation and handle correspondence. File and keep medical records up to date.

THE HIRING PROCESS

A cheerful office assistant, one with tact and understanding and who is efficient, can be an important asset to your practice as well as relieve you of the burden of a myriad of details. It will be well worth your time and trouble to hire a person you can work with who has the qualities you desire.

Recruitment

Your first step in recruiting an office assistant might be to talk to the people you know, both socially and professionally, and let it be known you are looking for an assistant. Call the personnel director at the hospital. He or she might know of a trained medical assistant who is looking for part-time work with a private employer who would be more flexible about hours than the hospital. Other professionals may know of past employees whom they could recommend who perhaps have retired to raise a family and are ready to come back into the job market on a limited or even a full-time basis.

If you need someone full time, look into the medical assistantship programs sponsored by the American Medical Association and the American Association of Medical Assistants at over 100 community colleges. These programs teach basic office skills and some clinical training. You can contact the AMA at 535 North Dearborn Street, Chicago, Illinois 60610 or the AAMA at 1 East Wacker Drive, Chicago, Illinois 60601. Your county medical or dental association may have a placement service or know of some well-qualified people.

Chances are that you will more likely find an appropriate person via the private route than by an open ad in the Help Wanted section of your local newspaper. However, if you are not able to wait for the right person to call you, word your ad carefully. Rather than call for a receptionist/secretary/bookkeeper or a "Gal Friday for a health practitioner," it is advised that you define the duties and forget the labels. For example:

> Assistant needed in health practitioner's office. Answer phone. Make appointments. Some correspondence and billing. Good typing. Some medical experience.

If you do not want the phone to ring every 10 minutes, have the applicants write to a box number at the newspaper office. This will screen out those who are too impatient or cannot write a proper letter. However, including a phone number in the ad gives you the advantage of immediately screening an applicant over the phone.

The "go no-go" telephone interview

Before making an appointment for a personal interview, ask some pertinent questions over the phone. This will give you a sample of the applicant's telephone personality. But more important, you will be able to settle the nuts and bolts issues with the applicant.

For a part-time office assistant you might ask the following questions:

1. Are you able to work 10–3 Monday, Tuesday, Thursday, and Friday, 9–5 on Wednesday? Or can we work out a modified schedule satisfactory to both of us?
2. Are you available year round?
3. Is _____ dollars per hour acceptable?
4. How many words a minute do you type? (55 would be satisfactory.)
5. Have you worked in a medical office before? (You are looking for a minimum of a year's experience.)
6. Have you experience in billing and bookkeeping?
7. Are you familiar with dictating equipment?
8. Do you have professional references?

If the answers to the preliminary screening questions are favorable and you find the person has a pleasant telephone presence, "go" for a personal interview and set up an appointment. You don't have to see everyone who responds favorably. You can put them off with the "Don't call me, I'll call you" routine. But take the person's name and phone number. The other candidates may fall through.

The personal interview

When an applicant arrives at your office, ask her/him to fill out an application. A uniform application gives a point of reference for comparing several applicants. You will want to accept and read people's résumés if they offer them, but bear in mind that résumés are self-serving. An application should ask for certain fundamental information, including a job history. Ask the applicant to sign the application attesting to the truth of the statements made. In the event that the person has misrepresented her/his job history, you will have a reason for discharge.

Application forms can be obtained at a stationery store or write your own form (see Figure 4–1).

An interview should be structured and open ended. That is, you should know what questions you want to ask, but allow the applicant to do a lot of the talking, even if not directly relevant to the question you asked. This will allow you to form an impression of the candidate's manner and intelligence. A good plan is to use the application and/or the résumé as a basis for the discussion. As you listen to the applicant, remember that this person is going to represent you to your patients. Is the applicant friendly and interested? Suspicious? Unable to hear your questions. Most patients call because there is something wrong. A patient may be anxious. You will need someone who has good judgment and kindness with an ability to listen and understand. You might want to draw up your own list of what you expect from an employee and present it as a part of the interview. You will also discuss the job description.

As an important part of the interview you will want to present the challenging and positive aspects of the job. A good applicant may have other possibilities and you may have to sell the job. You may find yourself telling the applicant about that part of your practice that you find rewarding and exciting. You will also use the interview to explain your personnel policies and benefits package.

The interview is a two-way discussion. The applicant will want to know about certain conditions on the job, and will be sizing you up as a prospective boss. Be candid and remember that you and the activity in your office will constitute a major part of the candidate's life. You will want to hire the candidate who will find working for you and your patients rewarding and satisfying.

Take notes on each interview. If you discuss salary and hours, be sure to keep track of what you have agreed to. After talking to four or five people you may mix up what you said to whom.

References. Do not hire an applicant on the spot. You will want to call at least one, if not more, of the professional references indicated to verify a candidate's story. Ask the reference specific questions. When did the applicant work for you? What duties were performed? Why was the relationship terminated? Was the person good at her/his work? What about punctuality and attendance? Would you rehire the person? Then you might ask for an overall impression such as, was this person a valuable employee and did you like the person?

PERSONNEL POLICIES

An employer cannot be casual about benefits, holidays, vacations, raises, and other personnel matters. These policies are going to govern the conditions under which your employees work. You must be explicit and they must understand the policies so that you and they can act accordingly. Put together a personnel policy manual (it may not consist of more than one or two pages) and include it as a part of your contract of employment.

FIGURE 4-1

APPLICATION FOR EMPLOYMENT

PERSONAL INFORMATION

DATE _____

NAME

SOCIAL SECURITY
NUMBER

LAST	FIRST	MIDDLE

PRESENT ADDRESS

STREET · CITY · STATE

PERMANENT ADDRESS

STREET · REFERRED · CITY · STATE
BY

PHONE NO.

EMPLOYMENT DESIRED

POSITION · DATE YOU CAN START · SALARY DESIRED

ARE YOU EMPLOYED · IF SO, MAY WE INQUIRE OF YOUR PRESENT EMPLOYER?

EVER APPLIED TO THIS COMPANY BEFORE? · WHERE? · WHEN?

EDUCATION	NAME AND LOCATION OF SCHOOL	YEARS ATTENDED *	DATE GRADUATED *	SUBJECTS STUDIED
GRAMMAR SCHOOL				
HIGH SCHOOL				
COLLEGE				
TRADE, BUSINESS OR CORRESPONDENCE SCHOOL				

* THE AGE DISCRIMINATION IN EMPLOYMENT ACT OF 1967 PROHIBITS DISCRIMINATION ON THE BASIS OF AGE WITH RESPECT TO INDIVIDUALS WHO ARE AT LEAST 40 BUT LESS THAN 70 YEARS OF AGE.

GENERAL

SUBJECTS OF SPECIAL STUDY OR RESEARCH WORK

WHAT FOREIGN LANGUAGES DO YOU SPEAK FLUENTLY? · READ · WRITE

U.S. MILITARY OR NAVAL SERVICE · RANK · PRESENT MEMBERSHIP IN NATIONAL GUARD OR RESERVES

SPECIAL QUESTIONS

DO NOT ANSWER **ANY** OF THE QUESTIONS IN THIS FRAMED AREA UNLESS THE EMPLOYER HAS **CHECKED A BOX PRECEDING** A QUESTION THEREBY INDICATING THAT THE INFORMATION IS REQUIRED FOR A BONA FIDE OCCUPATIONAL QUALIFICATION OR DICTATED BY NATIONAL SECURITY LAWS, OR IS NEEDED FOR OTHER LEGALLY PERMISSIBLE REASONS.

☐ HEIGHT _____ FEET _____ INCHES ☐ CITIZEN OF U.S. _____ YES _____ NO

☐ WEIGHT _____ LBS. ☐ DATE OF BIRTH* _____

☐ _____

*THE AGE DISCRIMINATION IN EMPLOYMENT ACT OF 1967 PROHIBITS DISCRIMINATION ON THE BASIS OF AGE WITH RESPECT TO INDIVIDUALS WHO ARE AT LEAST 40 BUT LESS THAN 70 YEARS OF AGE.

FIGURE 4–1 *(concluded)*

PHYSICAL RECORD:

DO YOU HAVE ANY PHYSICAL DEFECTS THAT PRECLUDE YOU FROM
PERFORMING ANY WORK FOR WHICH YOU ARE BEING CONSIDERED?

WERE YOU EVER INJURED?   GIVE DETAILS:

HAVE YOU ANY DEFECTS IN HEARING?   IN VISION?   IN SPEECH?

IN CASE OF
EMERGENCY NOTIFY

	NAME	ADDRESS	PHONE NO.

FORMER EMPLOYERS (LIST BELOW LAST FOUR EMPLOYERS, STARTING WITH LAST ONE FIRST)

DATE MONTH AND YEAR	NAME AND ADDRESS OF EMPLOYER	SALARY	POSITION	REASON FOR LEAVING
FROM				
TO				
FROM				
TO				
FROM				
TO				
FROM				
TO				

REFERENCES:
GIVE BELOW THE NAMES OF THREE PERSONS NOT RELATED TO YOU, WHOM YOU HAVE KNOWN AT LEAST ONE YEAR.

	NAME	ADDRESS	BUSINESS	YEARS KNOWN
1				
2				
3				

I AUTHORIZE INVESTIGATION OF ALL STATEMENTS CONTAINED IN THIS APPLICATION. I UNDERSTAND THAT MISREPRESENTATION OR OMISSION OF FACTS CALLED FOR IS CAUSE FOR DISMISSAL. FURTHER, I UNDERSTAND AND AGREE THAT MY EMPLOYMENT IS FOR NO DEFINITE PERIOD AND MAY, REGARDLESS OF THE DATE OF PAYMENT OF MY WAGES AND SALARY, BE TERMINATED AT ANY TIME WITHOUT ANY PREVIOUS NOTICE.

DATE   SIGNATURE

INTERVIEWED BY _____ DO NOT WRITE BELOW THIS LINE _____   DATE

REMARKS:_____

NEATNESS		CHARACTER	
PERSONALITY		ABILITY	

HIRED	FOR DEPT.	POSITION	WILL REPORT	SALARY WAGES

APPROVED: 1.   2.   3.

EMPLOYMENT MANAGER	DEPT. HEAD	GENERAL MANAGER

THIS FORM HAS BEEN DESIGNED TO COMPLY WITH STATE AND FEDERAL FAIR EMPLOYMENT PRACTICE LAWS PROHIBITING DISCRIMINATION ON THE BASIS OF AN APPLICANT'S SEX OR MINORITY STATUS. QUESTIONS DIRECTLY OR INDIRECTLY REFLECTING SUCH STATUS HAVE BEEN INCLUDED ONLY WHERE NEEDED TO DETERMINE A BONA FIDE OCCUPATIONAL QUALIFICATION OR FOR OTHER PERMISSIBLE PURPOSES, SUCH QUESTIONS ARE APPROPRIATELY NOTED ON THE APPLICATION. NOTWITHSTANDING THESE EFFORTS, THE MANUFACTURER OF THIS FORM ASSUMES NO RESPONSIBILITY AND HEREBY DISCLAIMS ANY LIABILITY FOR INCLUSION IN THIS FORM, OF ANY QUESTIONS UPON WHICH A VIOLATION OF STATE AND FEDERAL FAIR EMPLOYMENT PRACTICE LAWS MAY BE BASED.

Personnel policy manual

The following are some suggestions for policies that should be included.

1. This office does not discriminate because of age, race, religion, or sex in hiring personnel.

2. The first three months of employment will be a probationary period. At the end of this time there will be an evaluation during which employee and employer will discuss their mutual benefit to continuing the relationship. Medical insurance and other fringe benefits will commence at this date.

   (At the end of three months you can both sit down and talk about the job. If the individual does not seem to be working out, it is better to terminate at this point than to have an incompetent or unpleasant person in your office.)

3. There will be a regular yearly evaluation.

   (Sitting down again, maybe over lunch, can give you and an employee a chance to talk about ways to improve the office procedures or offer an opportunity for you to say how pleased you are with the general conduct of the office. It is a good time too for small complaints. If complaints are major, you might think about terminating the relationship.)

4. A policy on raises should be articulated.

   (Raises on a yearly basis for merit are important for morale and can be a part of the yearly evaluation.)

5. Cost-of-living increase.

   (With inflation, some attention must be paid to a cost-of-living increase. It is awkward for employees to have to ask for a raise. If you refuse, they have to seek employment elsewhere. Far better to offer a raise as an acknowledgment of your desire to continue the relationship. A good idea is to lock pay raises into raises in fees.

6. Benefits. Medical insurance, pension, dental insurance. If a person has worked for you for three years, you must include him/her in your Keogh Plan.

7. Holidays. Most health practitioners give their employees the customary six paid holidays: New Year's Day, Memorial Day, Independence Day, Labor Day, Thanksgiving, and Christmas.

8. Paid vacation. Vacation time varies from office to office from one week a year, for example, to one week after six months, two weeks after a year, and three weeks after five years.

9. Other paid days off. Some employers offer from 5 to 10 paid sick days. Some may give two or three personal days for an employee to conduct personal business.

Salary levels

How much to pay an employee may be a bothersome question. When you first open your office, you will be feeling strapped and will want to pay as little as possible. After your practice starts to grow, you will have less time to supervise your affairs and will want a more capable person. Salaries are a tax-deductible expense, so $5 or $10 a week will scarcely cost you anything.

There are several strategies you might pursue in establishing a starting salary. Far and away the best bet and the most honorable, is to pay the going rate. You might justify a low starting salary by pointing to the amount of time you will have to take from time spent with patients to show a new employee your office systems. A new employee who has worked for a health practitioner before will need only to learn the ways your routines differ. You might use the three months evaluation as a time to bring the salary up to the prevailing starting wage in your area. Or, if you start at the prevailing wage, you might wait until a year is up for the first raise. Experienced candidates will not work at less than the prevailing rate, although they might be willing to work for less during the three-month probationary period.

How can you tell what the prevailing wage is for a medical office assistant in your area? Ask others in your specialty what they are paying. You will also get a good idea of the prevailing rate from the applicants as you interview them.

Another strategy is to pay a lower rate but allow for greater flexibility in respect to hours. A woman applicant might be willing to take less pay if she knows that she can adjust her hours to accommodate her children's needs or if she will be allowed to take care of her family in case of an illness with no penalty. But you will have to do without her assistance when she is not available. At first a cheaper, flexible arrangement may seem attractive, but as your practice grows, you may find it inconvenient. On the other hand, hiring an individual who can fill in at odd hours may be an excellent arrangement for a second employee to do billing, filing, bookkeeping, and other nondaily chores.

Binding the agreement

It is good practice to put your verbal agreement into writing when you hire an employee. A written agreement makes the hiring of an assistant, even part time, appear as a less personal arrangement. It establishes a certain distance between employer and employee. The position becomes that of a worker or employee, not a servant. Perhaps more important even than establishing a professional tone to your relationship, a written agreement helps to avoid misunderstandings.

The agreement which can be written in simple nonlegal language in the form of a letter should include salary, hours, and the items just enumerated as personnel policy: paid holidays, vacations, raises, medical insurance, pension plan, and so forth. To make the agreement binding and to insure that both parties understand and are fully aware of the contents, it should be signed. The employee should be given a copy. Once you have worked out an employee agreement, it can easily be modified to suit other employees over the course of your career.

Hiring professionals

It is highly likely that you will sooner or later hire a professional as a consultant or a member of your staff—an oral hygienist, a psychological tester, a nurse practitioner, a part-time or full-time associate. Essentially the process is the same. Your main emphasis will be on keeping the arrangement businesslike and the duties explicit—they will perform a service for you and you will pay them. The principal way in which the process differs is in recruitment.

There are a number of ways for recruiting professionals. Word-of-mouth will probably give the best results. Talk about the kind of person you need to all of your colleagues when you see them socially or professionally. You no doubt have already learned how small a world is that of your own specialty—a world in which everyone knows everybody else and everybody else's business. If your own acquaintance does not yield a few candidates fairly promptly, write or call your local professional organizations and that of the specialty you are seeking. Keep a file of the letters and résumés people send you. It may seem almost silly to you now, but you may regret not having saved them later. Even if those people are no longer available, they may have a well-qualified friend.

Conditions of employment

How are you going to pay a professional. Your arrangements may run all the way from a fee charged by the professional, for example, for psychological testing, to a full-time salary with all the fringe benefits. This will be a matter of negotiation between you and the professional. Put your agreement in writing. Again in the form of a letter, the agreement should specify compensation as well as responsibilities and conditions. A sample letter is shown in Figure 4–2.

HOW DO YOU KEEP YOUR STAFF HAPPY AND PRODUCTIVE THOUGH WORKING?

Personnel policy does not end with a written statement of working conditions. The principal condition you will provide is an unwritten one—the atmosphere in which the work takes place. Your attitude toward your employees will be the chief ingredient. Do you think they are too slow, stupid, lazy, inefficient, contrary? Do you change your mind after a job has been completed and want it done another way? Do you ignore them completely except when you need something or can't find something? Do you treat them like children or servants? Do you reprimand them?

FIGURE 4-2
Sample letter of agreement

ROBERT M. DAY PH.D.
PSYCHOLOGIST
3 Bay Terrace
Middletown, Rhode Island 02345
401-333-1234

July 27, 1982

Mr. Jerry McLear, Ph.D.
41 Quanscutt Lake Road
Charlestown, Rhode Island 02334

Dear Jerry:

This is a letter agreement which will set forth our mutual understanding regarding the nature of consultation service you will provide to patients seen in my offices.

1. Duration.
The duration of this contract shall be for one year.

2. Presentation to the public.
While providing consultation services in my office, until you are licensed in accordance with Rhode Island State law, you will not be held out to the public as a "psychologist." You may be presented as a "therapist" or "psychotherapist" or any other descriptive term congruent with the State law of Rhode Island and with the Standards of Ethics of the American Psychological Association.

3. Consultation fee.
You will keep an accurate record of all consultations provided in this office. Reimbursement will be based on this record which will be your responsibility to keep current. Reimbursement will be provided as follows. Fees will be designated as either Type A or Type B. Type B fee will be paid for any patient who is charged less than 60% of the actual fee or from whom less than 60% of the fee might be anticipated. Type A fee will be based on any patient from whom 60% of the fee or more is anticipated. The only exception is that the consultation fee of $80 will be paid for any psychological evaluation or testing battery consisting of at least three to four hours in duration. An evaluation or battery will include presentation of completed protocol to me and will be considered complete when your report is dictated in final form. You will be paid regardless of whether or not the patient reimburses me. You must, however, have contact with the patient. In other words, you will not be paid if a patient does not show for an appointment. Group sessions will be paid at a one hour Type A rate. These sessions will entail both contact with the patients and pregroup and postgroup supervision. Type A consultation will be paid at a rate of $20, Type B at $15.

FIGURE 4-2 *(continued)*

4. Malpractice.

Your malpractice insurance liability is completely your responsibility. Although my own malpractice insurance may protect me from liability accrued in relationship to your work done in my office, it is not my responsibility to provide you with coverage.

5. Memberships.

You will maintain membership in good standing in the American Psychological Association.

6. Limitation of private practice activities.

During the duration of this contract, your private practice activities in Narragansett, South Kingstown, North Kingstown, and Aquidneck Island will be limited to consultations provided through the auspices of my offices servicing these geographic regions. This contract will not prohibit you from any employment with any public agency or educational facility, nor will it prohibit you from providing private practice activities and consultations as designated in Item 7 in the areas other than Narragansett, South Kingstown, North Kingstown, and Aquidneck Island.

7. Responsibilities.

Your consultations for me will be implemented by providing individual and group therapy to patients provided either by your own referral or mine. You will be prompt for appointments. You will also provide diagnostic work and maintain clinical records in a manner prescribed by me. For all visits you will also provide and produce reports as needed. You will be responsible for the collection of fees of those patients that you see and provide these patients with proper receipts. You may also be called upon to provide school visits and parent consultations. You will supply all material, devices, record booklets and test protocol. Transportation and other incidental costs will be born by you. I will provide you with office space, secretarial assistance, and with access to telephone and answering service.

8. Supervision.

Apart from specific consultation you provide me, I will make available to you and provide you with supervision regarding patients you see under my auspices in a manner consistent with good clinical practice and in a manner consistent with standards for practice promulgated by the American Psychological Association.

9. Conflict of interests.

During the extent of this contract, if you provide services for another employer or contractor as outlined in Item 6, you will be responsible for monitoring and preventing any conflict of interest that may be present to you as consultant to me and either as the employee or consultant of others. I will not be responsible for any allegation of conflict of interests in regard to multiple consultations or employment.

10. Termination.

Upon the termination of this agreement, you will not engage in any other private practice activity either for yourself or under the employ or as a consul-

FIGURE 4-2 *(concluded)*

tant to any other private practice agency or practitioner in Narragansett, South Kingstown, North Kingstown and Aquidneck Island for a six month duration.

If this agreement is satisfactory to you, please sign the original and return it to me, keeping a copy for yourself. My signature below along with yours will then consititute a letter of agreement between the two of us.

Sincerely yours,

Robert M Day

Robert M. Day, Ph.D.

I agree to the above terms.

7/29/82

Date

Jerry McLear

Jerry McLear, Ph.D.

RMD:sw

All of the above are no-nos. People sense an attitude even if unspoken. Think back over the jobs you have had since you were a teenager and the bosses or supervisors you have worked for. Were you fortunate enough to have had one or two who made the job interesting even if it was only piling boxes in a stockroom? Did you have a sense of participation? Can you still get a glow of accomplishment when you remember an improved method you thought of for doing something? Most people will give you their best if you show respect and appreciation, particularly if they are encouraged to think for themselves.

"Let others take care of the details." That is the advice of Stanley Wantola of the Small Business Administration. That means you have to let go of some of the management of your office. This is known as delegating authority. Delegate responsibility as well.

Here are some of the ways you can show that you consider an employee to be an intelligent, reasonable, responsible human being.

1. You have defined the work to be done in the job description. Allow the employee to decide how she/he will arrange the daily schedule and go about accomplishing the task. Ask some questions to make sure that the task is understood. Your job is to make that clear. You might explain how it has been done in the past. Some people like to be told. Later they may make their own modifica-

tions. Now stand back and let the wheels turn. If you see that the employee is going about the task slightly differently or following a different time schedule, that's OK, provided all the work gets done. It means the employee is involved and that's the most you can ask for your money.

2. Allow an employee to make mistakes. Making mistakes is integral to the learning process. An employee who was responsible for ordering the office supplies, ordered a dozen rolls of scotch tape at a bargain price. The tape was defective. She wrote a letter of complaint and got the money back. She was allowed to suffer the consequences of her judgment and rectified the situation.

3. Unless you are ready to fire the employee, avoid scolding, complaints, and other forms of reprimand. Reprimands are likely to frighten most people, or make them angry. Fear and anger do not improve most people's job performance. Most people know when they have made an error or have not performed as expected. Let them tell you. And let them tell you how they intend to rectify the situation.

4. Let employees do things they like to do. For example, an office assistant liked to go to the library to use the copier. It got her out of the office for 20 minutes or so and she came back refreshed and with some sense of control over her own work schedule. On a busy day, however, she might copy the correspondence on the way home, stuff the envelopes at the library, and choose a route home by way of the post office.

5. Encourage an office assistant to compose letters when they are of a non-clinical nature. Your request might be, "Tell Dr. Strangelove that I'd like to have lunch with him during the Miami conference." For correspondence that is not personal, the assistant might sign his/her own name, as for example, questions about billing or requests for information.

6. A practitioner may have unrealistic expectations of how much an employee can accomplish. Don't expect him/her to be a clone of yourself. He or she may not work as fast or as efficiently as you do. That is why you are the professional and the employee the assistant.

7. Set priorities. When things get hectic, what to you are the most important things to be done? What can wait? You cannot expect an employee to guess.

8. When you want something to be done, be explicit. Say what you want, allow for feedback, and reach a decision. The "by the way, why don't you, if you have a chance" request does not constitute a work order. They will respond literally. If you want something done, say so in a definite manner. "I want the December bills in the mail by the first of January. How are you going to handle it with the holidays?" You listen to the answer and come to an agreement. "That's a good idea. If the patient load is light, maybe we can all go home early during Christmas week."

9. *Don't dump on employees!* If you are having a fight with your spouse, you are anxious about a lack of referrals, or you can't handle all the patients you have, don't take it out on the nearest person at work. Yes, you pay them, but not to bear the brunt of your anger. An apology later does not make up for an outburst.

10. Try to avoid mixing your business life and your personal life. Be helpful and solicitous but don't get involved in the personal problems of your employees and don't confide in them about yours.

11. Don't advance money to employees. It makes you dependent on them since you will have to keep them on until the money is paid off. It also puts the employer in the position of being benevolent because you have it to give. It smacks, too, of the servant/master relationship.

12. You must not allow patients to intimidate office personnel. Your staff must be able to count on your support when disputes arise with a patient.

For your part, there are certain standards that you will set for employees. You are paying for their services and have a right to demand excellence from office employees. Letters should be spelled without errors. Names must be spelled correctly. Information taken over the phone must be explicit. There must be no errors in billing notices in respect to charges, names and addresses. And, above all, patients must be treated with respect and courtesy.

Supervision and control

Although you will be delegating authority to employees, it is essential that you keep control. After all, it is your office and you are the boss. You keep control by holding an employee responsible for completing assigned tasks and by checking to see that the job is done satisfactorily. The best way to check up is to have an employee responsible for making a report on a daily or weekly basis. It need only be a checklist if the tasks are routine. If you assign special tasks, write them down. Ask that they be included in the report.

Employees should keep time sheets and you should look them over. An attendance record should be kept. How else can you keep track of sick days, vacation, and personal days?

A regular daily or weekly meeting will give you a chance to make requests, set priorities, and check on work that has been done. A businesslike routine is to have reports read at the meeting. In the process of preparing a report, an employee will have to check over work that has been done, tie up loose ends, and attend to matters that have been let go in the press of more urgent things. It will force you, too, to gather together at one time the things you want done in your office. Thus a regular meeting gives a point of reference as well as a deadline.

There should be a sense of give-and-take at a meeting. You can involve your employees in some of the decision making—the arrangement of the waiting room, ways to save money on supplies, how best to handle the relatives of a patient. With an added sense of participation should come greater care in handling your affairs.

Regularly scheduled office meetings offer a forum for complaints on both sides. It is the time and the place for airing grievances rather than letting them slide by and accumulate.

The meeting need not last long. A daily meeting first thing in the morning may not go longer than 5 or 10 minutes; a weekly meeting not too much longer, depending on how many employees are present. If you expect your employees to be serious about their reports and the meetings, you must be too. Try not to let other appointments interfere with the meeting. Let the answering service take your calls. Take notes and keep a record of assignments, deadlines, and accomplishments.

CONFIDENTIALITY

There should be hard and fast rules about the rights of patients to privacy. Patients may have access to their own records but records should never leave the office. Employees must understand the issue of confidentiality. You might ask them how they would feel if they thought that their own doctor was talking about them as a case to his/her family or friends, or making jokes about their condition.

Patients should never be referred to by name out of the office. You should set the example by never referring to a patient except in the course of business, and never make jokes about patients. See Chapter 8, "Clinical Records and Other Professional Responsibilities," for a fuller discussion of confidentiality.

TERMINATION

When you fire or terminate an employee, there will be a financial settlement. Two weeks notice must be given. You may give an additional two weeks severance pay, depending on how long the person has worked for you. Try to make an amicable severance arrangement even if you have to be more generous than you would like. A private practitioner does not need an angry person out there in the community who can create all kinds of problems.

If a person is surprised at being fired, there is something wrong in the way you handled that person (unless he/she is hopelessly incompetent and shouldn't have been hired in the first place). An employee needs feedback. If you don't like the way a person is doing something, be explicit when you discuss it. You can say, "I would like the patient records to be filed immediately after they are used. Be sure to keep the latest information on the top." You might explain how important this matter is to you and what the consequences are if it is not done properly. If, for example, you are firing a female employee because she talks on the phone all day to her friends, you have to let her know that you know that is what she is doing and that it is not acceptable to you, if only for the reason that it ties up your line. If she continues, and you fire her, she can scarcely be surprised. Employees need realistic feedback.

They need ego-saving information, too. "I know that you are upset that your daughter ran away from home, but if you are to come to the office and expect me to pay you, you have to get your work done." You can be lenient for a day or two but finally give a warning.

FIGURE 4-3
List of do's and don'ts in employer/employee relationships

1. Don't dump on employees.
2. Don't mix business and private life.
3. Don't lend money to employees.
4. Stress the importance of confidentiality to your employees.
5. Pay salaries on time. If you are casual about paying, you are giving an employee permission to be casual about working. Send out IRS forms on time (W-2s). Be prompt in fulfilling any obligations you have to employees.
6. Employees should sign in and out on a time sheet. If they are doing an office errand, that is included as time worked.
7. Petty cash should be available so that an employee does not have to come to you for small amounts of money. Petty cash records with all receipts for items paid should be kept up to date.
8. The same person should not do accounts receivable and accounts payable. It gives them too much information about your business (how much money you make after expenses). It also avoids embezzlement.

5

Building a practice

BUILDING A PRACTICE

Where do patients come from? How do you get them to come to your office? How do you keep them coming when they are in need of your specialty? Building a referral network depends as much on good and tasteful promotion as it does on good clinical care. To get and keep patients coming to your office, you have to make yourself and your specialty visible to both the general community and the local medical community.

Each medical specialty has a different set of problems in making a practice visible. Essentially they can be divided into three groups. Dentists and such primary care practitioners as pediatricians, general practitioners, family practitioners, and nurse practitioners are directly accessible to patients. Patients may be referred by friends; they may have heard your name mentioned, seen it in the paper, heard you speak, or met you socially; in an emergency they may find your name in the Yellow Pages; or they might have asked a pharmacist or another medical practitioner. People are more likely to choose a particular medical practitioner if they have heard about him or her from several sources.

A second group might include mental health practitioners, heart specialists, orthopedic doctors—the more common specialties. Patients usually come to these practitioners via the referral route from other people in the medical field. But, again, the patient is more likely to become yours if he or she has heard of you. This group needs to keep a high profile in the general community but will find that keeping his or her practice visible to other practitioners, especially those involved in primary care, is an important element in building a practice.

The third group are the superspecialists. These are always called in by another physician. The orthopedist who specializes in hands or knees, the radiologist, the oncologist, are dependent on referring physicians for their patients. Members of each of these three groups will use different strategies but all will need to keep a high profile to build their practices.

In the advertising business the promotion of a product is often referred to as a campaign because a number of different strategies may be employed at the same time. A TV commercial, a contest, ads in various women's magazines, and a national mailing of a sample of the product may simultaneously be utilized to launch a hair conditioner, for example. All these are directed toward the same end: that of making the buying public aware of the new product. Your efforts to gain visibility in your community might be conceived of as a campaign—not just the mailing of an announcement that you have opened your office, but a number of different strategies. From a listing in the Yellow Pages to an advice column in the local newspaper—your campaign must be planned as carefully as a Madison Avenue agency plans for its clients.

However, care must be taken that your promotional campaign does not make you unduly conspicuous. Bear in mind that you are a professional and that a direct appeal for patients may be viewed as tasteless. Your stance should be that you practice a particular health specialty and that you are available to the community. The soft sell is preferable to the hard one. Remember, too, that you are a member of a community of professionals. Older members may frown on a too blatant campaign for business and these old-timers may constitute a major source of referrals. On the other hand, you must be assertive. Hiding in your office will not bring in patients.

Watch the style of some of the more respected practitioners in the community. If you are new, do not be afraid to discuss referral systems with other practitioners. The directors of local professional organizations can be most helpful about what is considered permissible and tasteful and what is criticized and thought to be too pushy in the community in which you practice. A second caveat relates to the way you handle patients after they come to you. No ad campaign can be truly successful with a product that is devoid of merit.

Perhaps the analogy of building your practice to the advertising tactics used by business is distasteful to you. The rationale for conducting a campaign to promote your practice is not that "everyone does it," although they do, but that it is an important and necessary part of being a professional. You have spent many years in training to take care of people who will need your services. The result should be a full appointment book and the opportunity to practice your skills. However, if nobody knows who you are and what are your particular areas of expertise, there will be no one seeking your services. Keeping yourself visible in the community is an aspect of your work which, alas, is not explicitly taught as a part of your training. People have to know, too, that you want referrals. They may mistakenly assume that you have all the patients you can handle.

The campaign

The word *campaign* originally referred to the total effort of a military commander deploying his forces in a number of different ways to win, not just a battle, but control of a geographic area. A campaign to promote yourself and your practice will consist of a number of different actions. The following is an account of a pedodontist who moved to a small town and opened an office in an area with a poor history for pedodontists (another dentist had maintained a branch office and closed it down). An innovative approach was indicated.

Dr. X planned a spectacular office, one to excite comment. This office was to be quite different from the traditional dentist's office with its tiny cubicles, each equipped with a chair and instruments. He opted for a trilevel space. Three banana chairs (each in a different primary color) occupied the highest level with no partitions so a child could see what was happening with the other children. No equipment was visible. A play area and reception room and office was on the middle level and the lower level designed for adolescents away from the little ones was more traditional with privacy for each patient. In the walls was a dispenser of helium for balloons as well as nitrous oxide for anesthesia.

In addition to the traditional announcements, Dr. X invited all the physicians in town and their families to an open house with wine and cheese at the new office replete with helium balloons. This was a nice way for a child to meet the dentist and for the dentist to meet the local doctors. He further exploited the novelty of his new office by arranging field trips for the kindergarten and first grades of the local school to meet a dentist and learn about the care of teeth. This, of course, became a yearly event. Another strategy was to apply to the school board to become the school dentist. Dr. X also advertised an emergency service available 24 hours a day—easy to do with an answering service (emergency patients turn into regular patients).

Dr. X managed to make himself highly visible and talked about and yet did not step over the boundaries of good taste. Although his office created a sensation, it was all in the interests of the children—the bright colors, the open plan, even the balloons could be justified in terms of preventing fear of dentists. This practitioner built his campaign around the innovative design of his office. He made himself visible both literally and figuratively. Everybody in town knew that a new children's dentist had opened an office. For the future he would need to keep in touch with the local pediatricians and family practitioners and maintain good relations with school officials.

Not many specialties lend themselves to such a conspicuous entry into the community. Most practitioners resort to a more conventional campaign in making themselves known to their colleagues, establishing a personal style and reputation, and maintaining ties with the other health practitioners in the community.

Basic strategies

Your most important goal is to make other health professionals in your community aware of you, of the particular specialty you practice and the population you serve, and to trust your competence. Second, unless you are a superspecialist, you will want to reach the wider public with the same message. The traditional strategies are: an advertisement in the local newspaper, if that is the practice in your community; a personal announcement; a listing in the Yellow Pages; and personal contact with local health practitioners. Regardless of whatever other innovative strategies you might try, none of these should be omitted, particularly making contact with other health professionals.

The newspaper ad.   In most communities it is standard practice for professionals to take a once-only ad in the local newspaper to announce that they are opening an office. Although theoretically the ad will reach the greatest number of people, it will probably do little more than raise the consciousness of your name and specialty for a limited number of people in the community. The local professionals will probably take notice of the arrival of a colleague when they see it in the newspaper. However, an ad is inexpensive and very little trouble. A one-time ad is also helpful if there is a change in your practice—if you move, take in a colleague, or add a specialty. The ad should be run only once because it is considered unethical advertising in most places to repeat an ad. Before placing the ad, it is best to check with the ethics committee of your local professional group.

The ad should contain your name, highest degree, office address and phone number, and opening date. You might add, "Hours by appointment." A newspaper will take ads over the phone, but to avoid any possibility of error, it is advisable to type your ad on your professional stationery and mail or hand deliver it to the newspaper office.

The size of an advertisement is expressed in column inches. For example, an ad that is two columns wide and runs down two inches is said to be four column inches. An announcement should not be larger than two columns wide and two or three inches down—four to six column inches. The people at the newspaper will know the size customarily run in your community or, if you are in doubt, consult your professional organization.

A typical announcement might read as follows:

Elizabeth Hornblower, R.N.
pediatric nurse practitioner and counselor to children and adolescents
announces the opening of her office at
3311 Bellevue Avenue
Oneida, Ohio 54321
208-772-4567
Hours by appointment

Announcements.   Mailing an announcement has the advantage of reaching a carefully selected target population of colleagues, local health professionals, and other referral sources. Neither an ad nor an announcement by itself will bring in referrals. However, the effect is cumulative. The ad plus the announcement are helpful in paving the way for a phone call or a personal visit. Many practitioners save the announcements they receive for future reference.

The announcement itself will contain the same information as the newspaper ad. The printing can cost from one to several hundred dollars depending on the quality of the paper and the printing method. The card stock should be of good quality and preferably plain white, with or without an indented area for the copy. Because setting up the plates and the presses is the major cost, there is little price difference between ordering 50 or 500.

The envelope can be written by hand or typed. But do not use address labels. They give the impression of junk mail. Use your return address because first class mail is returned to sender. This is a check on the accuracy of your addresses. An affixed postage stamp and a return address increase the likelihood that the letter willl be opened and read.

Mailing list.   Announcements should be sent to all possible referral sources in your area. It is always best to address announcements to an individual. The Yellow Pages of the phone book, although not the best source, usually contain names of all the physicians in the area. Also listed are pharmacies with the names of the proprietors and pharmacists. In addition, professional organizations usually provide or sell mailing lists. Or you can send announcements to physicians in care of the local hospitals. Mental health practitioners, nurse practitioners, dentists, and physicians with child and family practices will want to send announcements to school personnel who are in a position to make referrals: principals, assistant principals, special education directors, directors of guidance, guidance counselors, school psychologists, social workers, and attendance officers. Names and titles of school personnel should be available from the school office.

A directory of community services is available in most communities at the public library. Community directories include the names and addresses of most of the organizations offering a service in the community as well as the names and addresses of their directors. Directories usually can be purchased and are an excellent mailing-list source. In compiling your mailing list, do not overlook your own lawyer, your clergyman, family doctor, or dentist.

Your mailing list is one of the business assets of your practice. You will use this list for building your referral network. You might keep the names and addresses on 3 x 5 cards. Addresses and phone numbers should be kept up-to-date. Some people keep the spouse's name on their cards also. Note any contacts made with the person and the date of contact, referrals from the person, and any other pertinent information.

Personal letters.   Another direct mail technique is to write a personal letter to a potential referral source. Again you will want to pinpoint your target population which, for the most part, will be other physicians. Physicians are regularly sought out by their patients and others for advice on where to go for health care. Physicians still have the aura of father figures and their recommendations carry considerable weight.

A sample letter to a physician on your letterhead might read as follows:

Dear Dr. Stacey,

I have just opened an office on Bridge Street where I will be providing obstetrical and gynecological services. I hope my services may be of benefit to some of your patients.

I would be delighted to meet and discuss further with you the services I am providing.

Sincerely,

A suggestion to save you the trouble of typing each of these letters separately might be to have them photo copied. Many copiers will print your letter on supplied letterhead stationery with good results. Then you need only insert the date, salutation, and signature. The letter will appear to have been personally typed on your own letterhead. A business card may be enclosed. As with any form of announcement, attention must be paid to ethical considerations. The letter should be sent only once and only to referral sources, not to potential patients.

Brochures. A fairly common practice in some specialties is for the practitioner to work up a brochure that either describes the particular practice or is in some way educational for a referring source. A nurse practitioner, for example, might use a brochure to explain exactly what it is that a nurse practitioner does to help a patient. That is, under what circumstances one would refer a patient to a nurse practitioner. A psychologist might want to explain his or her specialty, anorexia, for example, and include some of the symptoms.

Figure 5–1 presents the brochure of a psychologist specializing in children and adolescents:

FIGURE 5–1
Brochure for a mailing

Robert M. Day
3 Bay Terrace
Middletown, Rhode Island 02345
401-333-1234

BASIS FOR PSYCHOLOGICAL REFERRAL

Child	*Adolescent*
1. Prolonged poor school performance, particularly if onset was sudden.	1. Immediate referral if suicide is referred to.
2. Nightmares for more than three weeks.	2. Poor school performance with a sudden onset.
3. Hyperkinetic reaction—organic or functional.*	3. Withdrawing reactions.
4. Poor relations with peers.	4. Where drug or alcohol is involved.
5. Unable to be "managed" by parents.*	5. Sexual difficulties, including pregnancy.
6. Phobic reactions, including school phobia.	6. Explosive personality or over-aggressive reactions.

*Likelihood of family therapy indicated.

Reverse side of brochure

REFERRAL PROCEDURE

Children

1. Have the patient's parent or guardian call the above number.
2. Dr. Day will personally arrange an appointment for your patient.

Adolescents

1. At your discretion, either the patient or his/her parents may call for an appointment.
2. Adolescents who call on their own for an appointment will be seen by Dr. Day without their parents for the first interview. Parent involvement will be discussed at that time.

In addition to its educational value, the strategy of the brochure is again that of a reminder. You write a note and enclose the brochure. The referring source will keep the brochure for further reference and it will be a reminder of your practice. Or, if you make a personal call, you leave a brochure.

Brochures are often printed on 8½ by 11 sheets folded in thirds to fit into a legal size envelope. One section is left blank for a name and address so the brochure can be stapled and used as a mailer. Your business-card information is printed on the front fold with descriptive material (your message) inside.

Direct contact

Once the health community is made aware of your presence, you have to make yourself stand out in the mind of the person who is making a referral. You may be remembered because of an article you wrote; the referring source may think of you because she saw you in the hospital cafeteria the day before; because your office is situated close to the patient's home; because someone mentioned you recently in a conversation; or you look like the person's brother. Some of these things you can control and some you cannot. However, there is no substitute for direct contact—a one-to-one meeting with another physician. Even a voice over the phone does not carry the same impact on a referral source as an actual encounter with the real person.

Since a meeting with a physician may last from 30 to 60 minutes plus travel time, care should be taken in selecting referral sources with whom you want to have direct contact. Try to see physicians who are not in competition but whose patients might be in need of your specialty. Younger physicians whose referral patterns are not so firmly established may be a better bet for a beginning practitioner than the older person with a set pattern for referrals. You will, of course, want to know and be on friendly terms with your competition. They will be your best source of information concerning both clinical matters and those pertaining to your practice and the community.

Your strategy in contacting a physician should be as straightforward as possible. Since it is advantageous for physicians to be well acquainted with the available resources in their community, don't think that you are imposing on the doctor's time. Most will welcome the opportunity to talk to you and get a feel for the kind of practice you are engaged in. A doctor will not see you if he or she does not want to.

Call to make the appointment. Don't beat around the bush. Be brief and clear. Here are some rules for presenting yourself on the telephone that you might keep in mind.

Basic rules for presenting yourself

1. Speak to the doctor. Don't leave a message other than your name and that you will call again. Don't try to have the doctor return your call. If you don't succeed in reaching the doctor after a couple of calls, give up.

2. "This is Dr. Zorin calling for Dr. Smith. Is he (she) available?" This message works. It is the most effective statement and gets results.
3. Introduce yourself, briefly explain your medical specialty, and indicate you would like to have a meeting with him or her.
4. *Always* use some tie-in. A mutual acquaintance has suggested you call or you have an interest in common.
5. Be fairly assertive and direct. Don't conclude the conversation without pinning down a time and a place for a meeting. End the conversation by repeating the time and the place of the meeting.
6. The best place to meet is your own office. Your office lends substance and reality to you as a medical practitioner. You might use some special equipment you would like to exhibit as an enticement. The other doctor's office is the least desirable. The atmosphere is distracting because of the phone and the press of business. Any neutral ground is satisfactory.
7. There is no harm in saying that your purpose is to receive referrals. When one practitioner was asked why he wanted a meeting, the caller, somewhat taken aback, blurted out, "Because I want you to refer patients to me." To the caller's surprise, the physician agreed to a meeting and eventually became a reliable referral source.

Your meeting with another professional need not be lengthy. It is what you say that counts. A certain amount of small talk greases the conversational wheel. But don't be afraid to come to the point. "I want your business. I am good. I have some openings for patients (if, for example, you are a psychotherapist). I am building my practice." You will probably come across best to another professional when you talk about what you do. It is what you know best—what you do, how you do it, your patient population, the concern you have for your patients, the courtesy you show them. You want to give assurance that your treatment will not reflect badly on the referring source.

In addition, you should provide the referral source with information about your training, orientation, and preferred clientele. Ask how much feedback the referring source requires concerning his or her patients. Most important, some format for referrals should be established. Some doctors like to have business cards of practitioners to whom they refer patients. You can indicate that you will send the doctor some cards, thus affording the opportunity for another contact. In any event, you should not be embarrassed about handing out a card.

Joining a hospital staff

The fastest and easiest way to develop physician contact for those practitioners such as psychotherapists, nurse practitioners, social workers, and other professionals who are not physicians and might not otherwise do so, is to join a hospital staff. Many diverse kinds of health professionals are incorporated into hospital staffs. Although they may not be granted full staff privileges, they will get good exposure to the local medical community.

The typical hospital staff hierarchy is as follows:

Active medical staff with full voting privileges regarding hospital policy is usually composed of physicians and dentists who have passed a probationary period.

Associate medical staff have all the qualifications and most of the privileges of the active staff but is comprised of new members who usually remain at the probationary status from one to three years.

Affiliate staff, consulting staff, or *courtesy staff* are honorary designations with limited privileges that seldom include admitting or voting. This status might entail such obligations as attending staff and departmental meetings and performing or being available to perform specific services at the hospital at certain times.

For physicians there is no question about the necessity of hospital staff membership. However, mental health practitioners, nurse practitioners, and other health practitioners such as physical therapists should become affiliated in whatever way they can with a hospital. Even if the practitioners do not enjoy full privileges and responsibilities, they become known to the medical staff at meetings and other hospital functions, including social ones. Certainly, questions regarding credentials are quickly laid to rest since credential review is necessary to become a staff member in any capacity.

Applying for membership. The first step is to write a brief letter to the administrator or medical director of the hospital indicating a desire for affiliation. The response to that letter will include some explanation of the hospital staff and structure and application procedure and materials. Usually the application is given first to a specific department for review. The application then may go to a credentials committee, an executive committee, and finally to a full staff meeting for a vote. Usually there is an interview before the final vote.

Since one of the values of hospital affiliation is the exposure it offers for other physicians to become acquainted with your skills, attendance at various meetings becomes an important strategy. Try also to spend a little extra time at the hospital, if you can. Eat lunch there or arrange to meet people there. You will be seen. There is always the possibility of chance encounters that will raise your visibility. Give some consideration to conducting a hospital workshop or continuing education program to familiarize others with your areas of interest and expertise. These will be advertised and your name and specialty will be seen by many more people than those who actually attend.

Contacting school personnel

It is customary to have meetings with school personnel at the school. Many school officials feel that employees are not working unless they are in school. Meeting in the school cafeteria is definitely not recommended.

When contacting school personnel, respect the hierarchy and regulations of the school. Unless you already know a referral source there, your first contact should be with the school superintendent.

In the initial conversation you should identify yourself and your profession, indicate that you have opened an office nearby, and request a meeting. The superintendent may provide the name of someone with whom he feels it more appropriate for you to meet, for example, the school nurse.

From this point on your contact will be with the person indicated by the superintendent. Although it is rare for a superintendent to be involved in referring students, protocol requires that he or she be contacted prior to contacting any other staff person. Similarly, you should contact the principal of a school before talking to any of the staff.

Unless instructed otherwise, you should *always* check in at the school office first when making a visit. Schools do not want strange adults walking around. At some schools you will be expected to sign in and out. During the initial visit it is both polite and instructive to ask for a tour of the building.

Other sources

Other sources are a medical base, correctional facilities, churches, homes for the aged, nursing homes, self-help groups such as Alcoholics Anonymous, Parents without Partners, Women's Centers, and Visiting Nurse Associations. Each agency or group will have its own idiosyncrasies. Continual contact with a group in which you are genuinely interested frequently results in referrals.

Communication with other professionals

As has by now become obvious, it is most important that you ask new patients the name of the person who referred them to your office. You need that feedback and you will want to acknowledge the referral. It is common courtesy to write a note of thanks, or, if you feel more comfortable, make a phone call to thank the referring source. If one person has referred a number of patients, you might take him or her out for cocktails or dinner.

Just as important as the thanks, is the feedback you give to the referring physician. Take care in handling a patient from another practitioner. Of course, make no comments except the most complimentary concerning the referring source. Respond promptly to the referring source with a call to see what has happened after you have seen the patient and follow up the call with a letter giving all pertinent information such as tests results, or your plan for treatment.

Any written communication from your office should be executed with care and courtesy in clear and concise English. Your communications filed away in other people's offices represent you. They are a visible testimony to your clinical competence as well as your integrity and professionalism. Showing your appreciation for referrals and prompt and professional feedback tells referring physicians that you handle their patients with care, courtesy, and expertise. It is the best advertisement for your services and likely to bring continuing referrals.

OTHER STRATEGIES

There are other strategies for building a practice to further the central goal of visibility, exposure, and personal contact. Some of these strategies are utilized by the insurance salesperson and other local businesspeople as well as other professionals, but that does not lessen their value. For example, become a member of such organizations as a church or synagogue, or a golf, tennis, or yacht club. Go to the meetings. Again, it is the personal contact that is important. Join civic and charitable organizations such as the United Way, but only if you intend to participate. A poor showing is worse than none. Local organization membership is more important for primary care practitioners than for those who get referrals only from other professionals.

There is an increasing interest in workshops of all kinds. A fee can be charged which can supplement your income. If your specialty or subspecialty lends itself to the education or training of others, put together a program for a workshop. Try to get sponsorship from a local organization or self-help group. All kinds of health-related issues lend themselves to workshops—alcoholism, cancer care, the hospice movement, diet and nutrition, the care of the elderly, of handicapped children, sleep problems, and myriads of self-help, growth, and self-improvement topics.

Similar health-related topics lend themselves to talk shows on television or radio. A psychologist and a dentist worked out a program to help people overcome their fear of dentistry. In conjunction with the workshop, they approached their local radio station:

Mr. Phil Donegal
WABCD Radio
140 Thames Street
Springfield, Massachusetts 12345

Dear Mr. Donegal

Dr. Heacock and I will be giving a workshop and seminar to help people to overcome their fear of dentistry. We thought that the discussion of these matters might make for an interesting program. I have enclosed an article from the *Daily-News* and will be calling you in a few days to see if you would be interested in pursuing this matter with us.

Sincerely,

Albert Hawley, Ph.D.

Note that this team of a dentist and psychologist snowballed their workshop and seminar into a newspaper article as well as a possible radio program. It is important to remember, lest you judge such a request as aggressive and self-seeking, that the local newspapers, magazines, radio, and television stations are always on the lookout for subjects for articles and programs. It is a no-lose situation. Everyone benefits.

Health professionals can themselves conduct regular columns in the newspaper. Their names become known to the public and other professionals in this way. In fact, this strategy works so well that columns can be bought from a service for this purpose.

You can offer to give free talks on your specialty for local organizations. Many community organizations have regular meetings with speakers. Find out who the program chairman is for the group. You will be welcomed as a speaker if your particular subject is of general interest or is compatible with the purpose of the group.

A news release about a talk or workshop should be submitted to the local paper. The release should include information about the program and the speaker's role in it. Such visibility may stimulate interest in other programs and have a cumulative effect on potential referrals.

6

Income

Does a discusssion of money make you uncomfortable? Do you close your mind to such concepts as cash flow, billing, and collections? Do you prefer to leave such matters to your accountant? If that is truly the case, private practice may take on a financially mysterious, perhaps even unmanageable aura, one which makes working on a salary for someone else an inviting prospect. If you take a certain pride in understanding accounting practices, in seeing to it that patients pay for your services, and in supervising the financial aspects of your practice, then you will be able to enjoy the freedom of the independent entrepreneur. Either way, familiarity with fundamental business techniques and rules are essential for maximum financial return for clinical efforts expended in a private practice.

You should be able with a quick glance at your books to answer such questions as: how much income has been collected this week? this month? this year as compared to last year? How many receivables are still outstanding? who owes them? and how are you going to collect? Medical practitioners today must also be knowledgeable about medical insurance and what is covered by the various plans, as well as being experts in the procedures involved in collecting fees from insurance companies and the various government agencies. Well-kept financial records are your protection in the case of a tax audit. In this chapter we will tackle the issues involved in keeping track of income and making sure that it comes in.

ACCOUNTS RECEIVABLE

Accounts receivable is the actual accounting record of the money you are owed and the payments received. It tells you how much money you have made. Since this information is basic to your medical practice, you will want a quick and easy means for keeping this record. It is recommended that you invest in a so-called one-write system for this purpose. There are several on the market but all work on the same principle—a system of forms with carbon-reproducing strips that allow you to make a record of each transaction in several key places. The system we will describe consists of a patient ledger card, a day sheet or log, and a transaction slip. The same entry will appear on each form and may also be reproduced for billing.

Patient ledger card. This form keeps a running record of all the financial activity of a single patient account, including services rendered, charges and payments, and relevant dates. The record substantiates billing. It may also be used in court as evidence of services rendered. It is often a more accurate record of patient contact than case notes.

The patient ledger card in a typical one-write system is divided into columns for date, patient's name, services rendered, fee, credits, and balance (Figure 6-1). The codes for services at the bottom of the card are used to simplify billing. The card may be photocopied and mailed in a windowed envelope for billing purposes.

FIGURE 6-1
Patient ledger card in a one-write system

STATEMENT

ROBERT M. DAY, Ph.D.

3 BAY COURT
MIDDLETOWN, R.I. 02345

TELEPHONE
401-333-1234

CHARGES OR
PAYMENTS MADE
AFTER LAST DATE
SHOWN WILL APPEAR
ON YOUR NEXT
STATEMENT

◄ BALANCES BROUGHT FWD. ►

DATE	CODE	INSURANCE				PREVIOUS BALANCE	PATIENT		
		CUSTO FEE	ANTICI FEE	PAYMENTS	NEW BALANCE		CHARGES	PAYMENTS	NEW BALANCE

SAFEGUARD FORM NO. LS-M4 S/C 12360C
IT IS ANTICIPATED YOUR INSURANCE
WILL PAY THE LAST AMOUNT IN THIS COLUMN

PLEASE PAY THE LAST
AMOUNT IN THIS COLUMN

DI—Diagnostic Interview
IT— Individual Psychotherapy
GT—Group Psychotherapy
FT—Family Psychotherapy
PT—Psychological Testing
1 H—One Hour

FKA— Failure To Keep Appointment
C—Consultation
SC—School Consultation
HC—Hospital Consultation
ROA— Received on Account
90 M—Ninety Minutes

FIGURE 6–2
Transaction slip in a one-write system

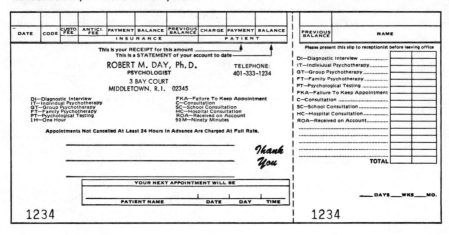

Transaction slip. The entry to the patient ledger card is repeated on the transaction slip (Figure 6–2). This is a disposable form given to patients which indicates to them the services rendered and the charges. If they pay at the time of the visit, which is most desirable, the transaction slip can be used as a receipt. It is also the form patients may submit to an insurance company or the Internal Revenue Service as proof of medical services received. You may give a billing envelope to the patient with the transaction slip if they do not pay at the time of the visit, to encourage prompt payment.

Day sheet. The entries for each patient will, finally, be reproduced on the day sheet (Figure 6–3). The day sheet provides a chronological account of all transactions and, as such, can be "proved" or balanced. It is a day-to-day and month-to-month record of accounts receivable. The three forms are kept in a special ledger designed so that each transaction is recorded simultaneously in all three places. This is your basic record for collecting money for services rendered and it spins off a financial record for each patient visit.

Every transaction must include the patient's name, the date, the type of transaction and fee, amount paid, and the current and previous balance. The day sheet used for illustration shows that Mrs. Chaves came in for a check-up and paid $15. She had no previous balance. Mrs. Carney on her initial visit was charged a $30 fee which she paid. Mr. Sprague mailed in $50, reducing his previous balance of $80 to a current balance of $30. To prove out the totals use the following formula found at bottom right of the day sheet:

$$\text{Columns } E + A - B - C = D$$
$$80 + 45 - 95 - 0 = 30$$
$$30 = 30$$

FIGURE 6-3
Day sheet in the one-write system

Day Sheet

DATE	DESCRIPTION	FAMILY MEMBER	A TOTAL FEE	B CREDITS PAYMENTS	CREDITS ADJ.	C D CURRENT BALANCE	E PREVIOUS BALANCE	✓	NAME	TRANS-ACTION NO.
									← Carry forward from today's totals only if more than one page is used today →	
9-2	Check-up		15 –	15 –		–	–		Mrs. Clever	1
9-2	Initial Visit		30 –	30 –		–	–		Mrs. Carney	2
9-2	ROA			50 –		30 –	80 –		Mr. Sprague	3
										4
										5
										6
										7
										8
										9
										10
TOTALS			A 45 –	B 95 –	C	D 30 –	E 80 –		Carry forward to top of next page only if more than one page used today.	

THIS PAGE OR TODAY'S TOTAL →

← PREV. DAY MONTH-TO-DATE TOTAL

↓ MONTH TO DATE TOTAL

PAGE PROOF OF POSTING
COL. E + A B C – COL. D

Form reprinted with permission from Safeguard Business Systems, 400 Maryland Drive, Fort Washington, Pennsylvania 19034.

FIGURE 6-3 (concluded)

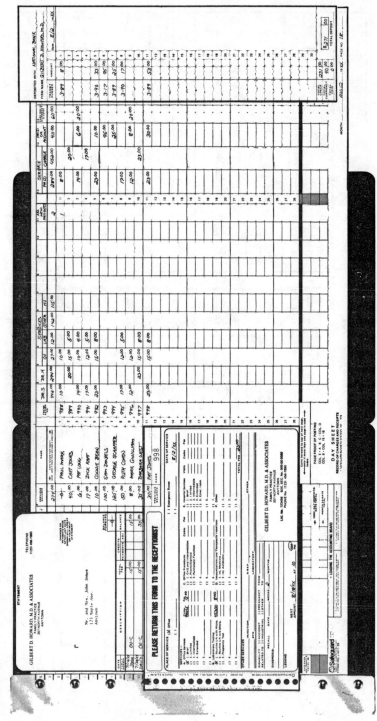

Form reprinted with permission from Safeguard Business Systems, 400 Maryland Drive, Fort Washington, Pennsylvania 19034.

Adjustments (adj. column C) are used when you do not expect a patient to pay the full fee. It is a way of showing the lowered fee or of writing off an uncollectible account. Entering the amount in the adjustment column removes it from the accounts receivable. A day-to-day review of accounts receivable is an easy matter with a day sheet. By not knowing who owes what, a practitioner can lose control of accounts receivable, that is, income.

Setting fees

Because of the prevalence of third-party payments, fees and categories of medical procedures are fairly well standardized. Practitioners set rates for each procedure; for example, an initial office visit, regular check-up, hospital visits, surgical procedures, lab tests, and so on. Rates for procedures are not set arbitrarily, but are determined according to what is considered a "usual and customary rate" (UCR). In today's inflation the UCRs for a particular area are based on statistics gathered by the major insurance companies which take into account all the rates in the area. Standard practice is to rank rates of practitioners with a formula that weighs the number of times a procedure is given, times the charges. Fees ranked at or below the 90th percentile are considered to be usual and customary. Some third-party payers such as CHAMPUS, however, limit reimbursement to the 80th percentile. Others determine the rates at which they will reimburse according to the individual profiles of each practitioner.

You can determine the local rates by writing Blue Cross and other large insurance companies that operate in your area. Sometimes a local professional organization will have results of a survey of rates or you can do your own minisurvey by talking to others in your field and asking what they charge. It is not considered an improper subject of conversation. In fact, most practitioners are only too eager to talk about fees.

It is recommended that even beginners set their rates at about the 90th percentile. It is much more difficult to raise your rates if you start too low. You can tell a referral source, "These are my rates. Of course, I always take particular circumstances into consideration. I don't turn people away." If you prefer to try for a higher volume, you can get into areas that pay less, such as Medicare or Workman's Compensation and lower your fees accordingly.

During inflationary times it is a good idea to raise your fees every year in accordance with the annual rate of inflation. Materials used, such as gold for fillings, might have to be raised in accordance with market considerations. When you raise your rates and it affects a long-term patient, do not forget to tell the patient about it, although some professionals do not make a change in their rates for ongoing patients. You may also want to inform old patients about rate changes when you see them again.

Many health professionals offer a courtesy rate to other practitioners. This may be experienced as a welcome surprise when a young practitioner with heavy family responsibilities is on the receiving end. However, it is not a universal practice. Practitioners will have to weigh the pros and cons for themselves.

Talking to patients about charges

It is always good policy to be open and direct about your fees. Never be apologetic. If a patient is going to be seeing you on a regular basis, for example, weekly sessions for psychotherapy, regular allergy shots, or prenatal visits, spend adequate time discussing the fee. Explain the services that will be included in the fee. A breakdown of the figures makes the total seem more credible. Dental services can be broken down into charges for each crown, for example, or lab costs. Discuss with the patient the way in which payments may be made (lump sum, monthly installments, etc.). It is possible to charge interest if the payments will be over a long term, but not recommended unless it has become standard practice in your area. Do not neglect to discuss the way you handle missed appointments, how much notice you require, making up missed appointments, and whether you charge for missed appointments not made up.

A discussion of fees offers the patient who can't afford to pay the full amount, the opportunity to say so. After you explain your fees you might say, "Will you have any problem with this? Let's talk about it and see if we can work something out." If the situation warrants, you may reduce the fee, although such exceptions should be rare. Your rate should be fair and equitable for 90 percent of the patients you see. Such a discussion is not a bargaining session. But it does allow you to hold to your established rates and yet be flexible with individuals. Spreading the charges over a period of time often lightens the burden.

Those who study the psychology of finances suggest that when patients make a payment to you or your assistant, look directly at them and thank them as you take the check. Look at the check, but not critically, and check the amount with a nod. This will convey the recognition that they have transferred money to you and that you appreciate it. If you take the check and stuff it in your pocket or toss it somewhere without even looking at it, you may be telling them that it is not important to you. And also that you may be a bit lax in your business arrangements.

If patients have an excuse about why they cannot pay, it is best not to help them along with the story or to convey sympathy. You will be letting them off the hook. But don't argue or show disbelief. However, if they "forgot the checkbook, it's in the car," don't be so anxious for the money that you make them run out to get it. In short, treat them with respect, but by your manner let them know that you are to be respected too, as is the agreement that you have together.

Agreements to pay. For long-term patients whom you will see again and again or for people who will owe large amounts, it is best to have a signed agreement. It makes clear the terms to which you and your patients have agreed. Often out of embarrassment or a sense of delicacy when dealing with both money and a medical professional on a first visit, patients will block out or not hear what the charges and the conditions are, even when you think you have explained them carefully. Ask them to sign an agreement such as the one shown in Figure 6–4. They will have it to look at and refer to later.

Practitioners who make arrangements with their patients for payments to be made in more than four installments must conform to the federal truth-in-lending laws whether or not interest is charged. The Figure 6–4 example contains the necessary information for compliance.

FIGURE 6–4

AGREEMENT TO PAY

_____(patient)_____ hereby agrees to pay ____(practitioner)____ ___(total fee)___ ,

less a down payment of $_____ , in 12 monthly installments of

$_____ each. The first payment will be made on ___(date)___ and subse-

quent payments on the first day of each consecutive month until the debt has been paid in full.

Total fee	_____
Down payment	_____
Unpaid balance (amount financed)	_____
Finance charge	_____(none)_____
Total cash price	_____

_____ _____
(patient's signature)   (date)

Missed appointments

For the busy primary practitioner with 8 or 10 patients in the waiting room, a missed appointment may come as a welcome relief, although some practitioners, in anticipation of "no-shows," may schedule more patients than they expect to see. A missed appointment, however, for dentists, specialists who put aside a half hour or more for a patient, and mental health practitioners, constitutes a financial loss. It is customary for dentists and psychotherapists to charge for missed appointments, but in actuality, it may be difficult to do so and keep the patient. The best most practitioners can do is to state a clear policy to that effect and try in every way to discourage missed appointments.

Discussion. Talking about missed appointments works as a deterrent. Make it clear that the hour missed is set aside for that patient. The psychotherapist can legitimately integrate the subject into a therapy session. If there seems to be a pattern of missed appointments, ask the patient if he/she is angry, afraid, etc.

Notices. Another deterrent is to state your policy in as many places as possible. For example, on the patient information form (see Clinical Records, Chapter 8) include a statement such as "Appointments not cancelled 24 hours in advance will be charged at the full rate," followed by "I have read the above statement and will honor this policy" and a signature. This message should appear as a sign in the waiting room and on patient's bills.

Procedures. Dentists routinely give the patient a card showing the date of the next appointment. Some dentists call each patient the day before an appointment as a reminder. The procedure has particular advantages in dentistry as appointments are sometimes given out six months in advance.

COLLECTIONS

The most advantageous way for a professional to collect fees is at the time the patient is seen. Some practitioners put up a discreet sign on the reception desk, "Payment expected when services are rendered." It saves billing costs and reduces risk of default. It has been estimated that a single bill can cost $2.50 to send out (postage, stationery, secretarial, and bookkeeping time). It also clarifies the situation on the spot if there is any misunderstanding about the amount or the balance due. Moreover, you have the immediate use of the funds. Bills sometimes don't go out for 30 days. You may not see the money for 60 or 90 days. That can represent a 2 percent loss or, if you are carrying a loan, a 3 percent loss. Also, patients who pay when they are seen or before they leave the hospital are more immediately aware of the service they have received and may be more willing to pay at that time. Patients who do not make regular visits are more likely to put medical bills at the bottom of the pile. The longer you wait for payment, the less likely you are to receive it.

Many medical practitioners use MasterCard or Visa. You are paid immediately by these credit companies. Collection is up to them. The fee charged you by the credit company depends somewhat on the size of the average "purchase" but it is usually in the neighborhood of 5 percent.

Facilitating payment

Probably you will find that at least half of your practice, if not more, involves third-party payments—people whose medical bills are paid by an insurance company or an agency of the government. And of the rest, many people will pay as they go or send a check promptly as they are billed. But there will always be those people who don't pay. Your first step in collection is to identify the people who have not paid.

A tickle system. A tickle system kept up-to-date is a daily reminder for you to do something—call or write—in this case about people who owe you money. Here is how it works. Use a box with 3 x 5 index cards and dividers numbered from 1 to 31. Each number stands for a day of the month. Notes to remind you about what to check on for a particular day can be placed behind the numbered card. Suppose Mr. Smith did not pay his January bill. On the first of February you will leave a reminder in the file behind card number 14 to call Mr. Smith. You or your secretary will check the tickle file every day. On February 14 you will call or write to Mr. Smith if his check has not yet been received.

Collection letters

Both the letter and the phone call are used in trying to collect overdue accounts. Since many people do not sit down on the first of the month and pay their bills, the first attempt at collection might be a written "reminder" followed by a series of stronger letters. Another strategy is to institute the phone call after a couple of letters have failed to evoke a response. The following series suggest the tone that might be adopted in collection letters:

First letter sent 45 days after first bill is sent out:

> Let me call your attention to the fact that this is the third statement you've received for the balance due on your account. If you have some question on the amount, or full payment isn't possible, please call so we can talk it over.

Followed by a somewhat less conciliatory:

> We don't know why you haven't contacted us on your overdue account. If you want to work out a payment schedule, please call. If not, please pay the balance in full.

The next is more urgent:

> Your account is very long overdue and some arrangement must be made immediately to take care of it. If there is a reason why you have not paid the balance, please call to talk it over. We must hear from you immediately.

And finally the threat:

> We haven't heard from you about your account although it is many months overdue. Since you don't want to make arrangements to start paying it, there is nothing we can do but turn it over to our collection agency. We will take that action in 10 days unless we hear from you. This is the last notice that you will receive from this office.

> (Ridgewood Financial Institute, 1980)

Noncontentious phone calls

Rather than wait for the person to call, you call. Consistent phone calls to speed collection has worked well for many practitioners. These can be made by you or your staff. A phone call might take place as follows: "I'm calling about your bill. I have noticed that there is a balance of $30." Pause for response. "Can it be paid by this Friday? Let me jot down a note to that effect. You will be paying $30 this Friday. Thank you. We look forward to receiving it."

Make a notation in the tickle file. If payment has not been received by Friday, call again. Their response is, "It's in the mail." Re-tickle it. Call back at work if necessary. When they say they have mailed it and can't imagine what has happened, you might ask them to stop by the office and drop off a check—"perhaps you can stop payment on the other check."

Don't argue. Be circumspect, polite, and don't question the credibility of their story. Above all, do not get angry. Once you show anger, you have lost the game and they have an excuse not to pay.

If you have reason to suspect that a patient is angry or unhappy with you or your bill, bring it out in the open. They may feel that you did not do anything for them, so why should they have to pay. Find out what the problem is and why they are angry. An angry patient should be handled carefully. Most malpractice suits arise out of some discontent with the bill.

At some point you may decide to make an adjustment to the bill. It is a better policy to persuade a person to pay a smaller amount and feel you are benificent, than to rigidly pursue an angry and possibly litigious patient.

Some people may be caught up in a temporary situation which prevents them from paying as, for example, loss of a job or a sudden extraordinary financial obligation. In such a case, you might come to an agreement with the patient. The Agreement to Pay form (Figure 6–4) is useful, specifying installment payments to commence when the personal crisis is over. Have the patient sign it.

Collection do's and don'ts

1. Keep an accurate record of each and every time you contact a patient on, or attached to, the patient's ledger card. Mark down all dates and amounts promised. There is power to the record. A patient quickly learns that you are not going to forget and that you will call when promised payments are not forthcoming.
2. Always be polite and listen. Don't interrupt. Always indicate the need for the bill to be paid. Get a commitment that the patient will pay a specific amount by a specific date.
3. Don't get into an argument or lose your temper. Don't threaten or say anything that you are not prepared to carry through.
4. Don't ask the patient "How much are you able to pay?" Better to say, "Can you pay the full amount by next week?" or if necessary suggest a specific amount as partial payment.
5. Always take the role of the understanding and kind person who expects to be paid.

6. Decide each case individually on its merits using a set of guidelines with which you are comfortable.

Pitfalls

"My insurance will take care of it." Patients may think they are covered, but it is up to the practitioner to ascertain whether, in fact, a patient is covered and what is the extent of the coverage. You or your staff will quickly become familiar with the terms of the contracts of the major carriers. Keep a code on each company with current information about rates and procedures. There may be deductibles and there may be maximums. Few people read the details of their policies. If you do not know about a particular insurance plan, you can ask your patient to bring in a copy of the policy.

Deductibles. Suppose you find there is a deductible or that the insurance pays 60 percent of the total bill. You might say, "Your insurance company pays 60 percent. All you have to pay is 40 percent." Or, "You only have to pay the first $50. The company will pay the rest."

Signing an agreement. Dental patients in particular seem to have trouble hearing or remembering just what work the practitioner said needed to be done and how much it will cost. If there is much work to be done, have them read and sign an Agreement to Pay as discussed earlier in the chapter and specify the work that will be included.

Bad risks. People and their children who are in the midst of a divorce situation may present problems in collections. The practitioner may be told that the father will pay the bill. Don't put yourself in a situation in which you are treating one person and expecting another to pay the bill. Make it clear in as nice a way as you can, that you expect payment from the patient or the parent who brings the child in.

Some practitioners find that people who miss their first appointment tend to be bad risks. Perhaps the ambivalence displayed by the missed appointment is still present when the time comes to pay the bill.

Psychotherapists find that court referrals and hospital consultations present poor credit risks in each case because the patients have not come of their own free will. It is easy for them to say, "I didn't ask for your services and I won't pay for them."

The bad debtor. Every practitioner must recognize that there are some people who are simply not going to pay. They enjoy getting away with it. They are skillful at nonpayment. Such people tend to be mobile and may even feign affluence. They come from every level of society. They tend to have the attitude that the world owes them a living. Most of these people are discovered after the fact. At the outset they may complain of financial problems. They may agree to pay every week and then soon begin to miss payments. This is a form of stealing, of course. Practitioners stuck with such a patient must make a decision whether and when to cut their losses.

Small Claims Court

If you decide to take legal steps to collect, the cheapest and fastest way is to use the Small Claims Court. The philosophy of Small Claims Court is to make it easy for ordinary citizens with no legal training to collect money they feel is owed them. The judge acts as a mediator, often suspending legal rules of evidence. Lawyers are not necessary. Usually you can get your case on the docket in six weeks or less and your claim is generally heard when scheduled.

When you go to court, take with you copies of the patient's ledger card, telephone record, and possibly your case notes. Present your case to the judge as follows:

1. Establish your credentials.
2. Give a record of your contact with the patient including the date when you were first called, the date when you saw the patient, treatment rendered, and the amount of the bill. Establish that the fee charged was "usual and customary." The patient did not pay. Technically, that is all the court will want to know.
3. If the patient presents a defense, as for example, "The doctor said the fee would only be X dollars," it will help to have evidence to refute the patient. Now is the moment to whip out your case notes. "We talked about the fee." The burden now is on the patient to refute your record.

If your evidence holds, you win the case. Winning the case, however, does not necessarily mean getting your money. The patient may default. You can go back to court and have the payment set up on an installment basis. If the money is still not forthcoming and the amount is sufficient to justify your time, you can file a lien against the debtor. Despite the propriety of your action, most practitioners would not go so far.

Using lawyers for collections. An alternative to Small Claims Court is to hire a lawyer. Most lawyers will not look at a claim under $1,000, but you might be able to find one who specializes in this kind of work and is willing to take on lesser claims. The first step the lawyer will take is to send out a "lawyer's letter" urging a patient to pay, with the implied threat or stated threat of a court proceeding. If you wait until you have a number of cases, the lawyer can take them all into court on the same day—a not too costly procedure. Keep in mind in choosing an attorney, that he or she will be your representative and a reflection of your practice.

Using a collection agency. Another alternative is to give your claims to a collection agency. Usually you will be charged from 25 to 40 percent of the funds collected, and no charge if nothing is collected. These people are apt to be pretty hardboiled and you might find that you do not want to be represented by them.

THIRD-PARTY PAYMENTS

Payments made to a medical practitioner on behalf of a patient by an insurance company or an agency of the government are known as third-party payments because technically speaking, the contract exists between an insurance company and the patient. When you accept assignment of payment, you become a third party to that agreement. Actually, there are several possible ways medical practitioners can be reimbursed by a company. They can, for example, refuse to accept assignment, as some doctors do. In such cases, the practitioner is expected only to provide documentation of diagnosis and treatment. The company reimburses the patient and it is up to the doctor to collect from the patient. In such a case, the doctor's fee is in no way controlled by the company.

If practitioners accept assignment, they bill the company and receive payment directly from the company. The patient must sign an agreement of assignment of payments to the practitioner each fiscal year. A practitioner may agree to accept the fee schedule of the company, in which case the patient may not be billed any further. Or a practitioner may accept assignment without agreement, not to be bound to the company's fee schedule, and bill the patient for the remainder of the fee.

Getting paid

The principal advantage for practitioners to accept assignment of third-party payments is that of actually receiving payment. The company or government agency expects you to present them with a clear documentation of who received the services, the patient's identification number, dates of service, type of complaint, and your charges. Some companies want you to use their forms, but most companies will accept the standard Health Insurance Claim Form. (See Appendix IV for Health Insurance Claim Form.)

Since, as mentioned before, you can expect to receive third-party payments from at least half your patients, it becomes an important matter to familiarize yourself with the regulations and procedures of the different companies and government agencies. For example, a practitioner billed an insurance company for treating "sexual disorders" for a couple who were having marital problems. When he had not received payment, he discovered that that company did not reimburse for treating sexual disorders. He resubmitted the claim form and changed the treatment to "psychotherapy."

In addition, there are informal arrangements that you should be familiar with. In one state, for example, according to the written regulations, psychological services are only covered by Blue Shield if the patient has been referred by a physician and if the psychologist is supervised by an M.D. Blue Cross discovered that the arrangement was expensive with the double fees. Furthermore, a court case in another state found against such a requirement. The rule still stands but it is ignored, an informal arrangement a psychologist in that state would need to be aware of. Participation in the informal network—lunching at the hospital, attending professional meetings, keeping in touch with colleagues—will help to keep you up-to-date with the vagaries of working with the insurance companies and government agencies.

Collecting third-party payments

The major problems in collecting third-party payments are in communications with the companies. Each item on the claim form must be completed to the satisfaction of the company. They will not pay until the paperwork meets their requirements. You can keep all the information concerning billings and payments on the two forms shown in Figures 6–5 and 6–6. The patient insurance activity form kept for each individual, shows at a glance the insurance identification number and the record of submissions and payments for that patient. The complete record for your follow-up on collections is shown on the monthly insurance submissions form.

Bill out the companies promptly. You might set up a system in which you bill out to a different company or groups of companies each week of the month—Blue Cross the first week, CHAMPUS the second week, and so on. Any bill that remains unpaid after six weeks warrants an inquiry. In Appendix IV you will find examples of letter forms which cover almost any problem you might have with a company. You should expect a prompt response to a letter. You can often cut through the red tape with a phone call, especially if there are questions involving dates of service or multiple family members whose names are confusing. A good rule is to send off a written inquiry after five weeks, followed up by a phone call after six.

FIGURE 6-5

PATIENT INSURANCE ACTIVITY					
Name:			Date of Birth:		
Address:			S.S. #:		
			I.D. #:		
Date submitted	Charges	Deductible	Due	Amount paid	Date paid

FIGURE 6-6

MONTHLY INSURANCE SUBMISSIONS

Date submit	Company	Patient	Dates of service	ID # and/or SS #	Profile	Deduc- tible	Amount due	Amount paid	Date paid

7

Expenses, taxes, and legal structures

EXPENSES
   Accounts payable and the one-write system
   The ledger
      Medical supplies
      Equipment
      Utilities
      Telephone
      Office supplies
      Rental services
      Repairs
      Auto
      Charitable contributions
   Filing systems
   Petty cash
FEDERAL TAXES
   The self-employment tax
   Paying taxes for employees
   What are your chances of an audit?
LEGAL STRUCTURES
   Sole proprietorship
      Advantages and disadvantages
   Partnership
   Corporation
   Which structure is best for your business?

EXPENSES

Expenses are the flip side of the bookkeeping record. A careful control over spending conserves what you have earned. And the record lets you know the extent of earnings over expenses—your profit. Even more important is the audit trail you leave for the Internal Revenue Service (IRS) since you do not pay taxes on collections which are turned around and put into the business. You are only taxed on the profit you have made. The IRS is particularly interested in the documentation you generate of the expenses you claim. Good records are also important because you may lose money by not claiming legitimate expenses for which you have no record.

Accountants complain that health practitioners do not take seriously enough the record of their cash flow. They also complain about handwriting that is illegible as well as incomplete records of expenses, particularly in such sensitive categories as entertainment and travel. Although English common law tells us that a man is innocent until proved guilty, it is the other way around when it comes to collecting taxes. In an auditing situation you are presumed guilty and must rely on the evidence of your records to prove that you have paid the government its due.

A cardinal rule of business is to keep personal and business finances separate. This applies to the checkbook as well. Corporations must by law maintain a checking account for the exclusive use of the business. All receipts from patients or other business income paid by check or cash must be placed in the business account, never in a personal account. No personal expenses can be paid out of the business account. Checks written to cash can only be for the practitioner's salary or draw. These rules are important not only to comply with the tax laws but for the practitioner's own records. How can you tell if the business is making or losing money or whether or not particular expenses are justified, if the record does not reflect the actual state of affairs?

The checkbook should be balanced each month when the monthly statement is received from the bank so that errors are picked up promptly. Cancelled checks must be kept for three years, the legal limit for a tax audit when no fraud is involved, but keeping them for seven years is a more prudent course. The checkbook (ledger), deposit slips, and cancelled checks lay down that all important audit trail for the IRS; that is, they provide the necessary evidence that documents and legitimates your business transactions.

Accounts payable and the one-write system

Since you will be paying for most expenses by check, consider a one-write checkbook which also serves as a double-entry ledger. The checks are bound into a ledger book. Each check features a strip of carbon paper running horizontally across the back which results in an automatic copy of the transaction onto the ledger. In addition to the checks and the ledger, the one-write system utilizes vendor cards. You can maintain a card for each vendor (a company or individual that provides goods and services). You slip the vendor card under the check. As you write each check, you are creating a record on the ledger and on the vendor card of the date of the check, the recipient, and the amount. You then enter the amount of the check in a designated ledger column, creating an itemized record of your daily, weekly, or monthly expenses. The ledger is your cash disbursement sheet and you will keep it by the month (see Figure 7–1). The vendor cards generate an audit trail by vendor. By subtracting each check as you go and entering deposits in your checkbook, you will be keeping a cumulative record of your bank transactions so that you will always know how much money you have in the bank. You generate this record every time you write a check.

The ledger

The ledger, bound into the one-write checkbook, enables you to record your expenses according to categories. You can obtain one-write checkbooks that can accommodate up to 18 columns for different categories of expenses. Whether or not a category warrants a column of its own depends on dollar volume and frequency of use. Remember you are creating a record for your own use, but more important, you are generating an audit trail for the IRS. Some categories are standardized by the IRS and you should use them, as for example: salaries, wages, etc.; rent; repairs, improvements, and replacements; depreciation; bad debts; travel, entertainment, and gifts; interest; insurance; taxes; and other or miscellaneous. The following are some categories for medical practice.

Medical supplies. These would include all consumable items, that is, supplies that are used up.

Equipment. Equipment includes all medical, office, and other equipment which has a life of over one year and that eventually wears out or becomes obsolete. The IRS calls this depreciable property and does not allow you to deduct the cost as an expense when you figure your business income for tax purposes. Instead, you depreciate it, that is, you spread the cost over more than one year and deduct it a portion at a time. Information about depreciation is contained in IRS Publication 334, *Tax Guide for Small Business*. However, if you borrow to pay for the equipment, the interest is deductible. Dentists, radiologists, and other medical practitioners who must invest in expensive equipment should consult an accountant to take the best advantage of the tax structure.

Utilities. These include heat, electric, gas, water, garbage collection, and fire protection.

Telephone. The Bell system is no longer the only company offering telephone equipment and service and they may charge the most in your area. Since it is expensive to change over once your equipment is installed, it may well be

FIGURE 7-1
D-11 disbursements

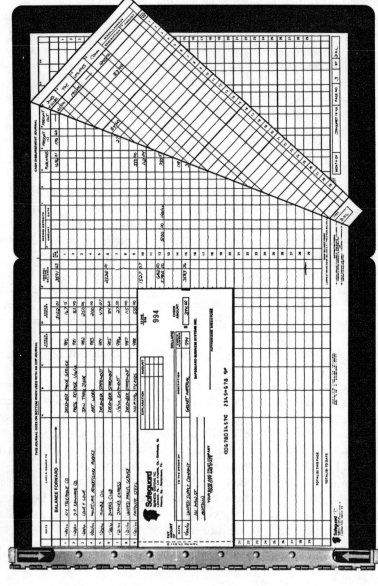

Form reprinted with permission from Safeguard Business Systems, 400 Maryland Drive, Fort Washington, Pennsylvania 19034.

worth your time to investigate competing companies as well as to inquire of the local Bell system about the varieties of services that might be appropriate for you. Be sure to ask about installation costs.

Office supplies. These are also consumable items, deductible as expenses.

Rental services. This category includes telephone-answering services, cleaning services, service for rental and maintenance of such equipment as a copier, typewriter, and medical equipment.

Repairs. If you own your own building, maintenance of building and grounds becomes an important item of expense. Painting, floor-waxing, and carpet cleaning would be included in this category. The IRS defines repairs as necessary expenses that do not add to the value of the property. Labor and supplies are deductible but not the value of your own labor.

Auto. The IRS permits you to take a standard mileage deduction. If you drive more than 4,500 miles a year, most accountants would advise you to take the deduction. If you have only one car, the IRS will not allow the full expense since personal use of your car is not a business expense.

If you choose to take the mileage deduction, you must, of course, keep track of your mileage. Many cars have odometers that can be reset. Keep a notebook in the glove compartment and post mileage every day. Currently, you are not allowed mileage between your home and your office but the mileage between two offices, from office to consultation, or from home to workshop is allowable. Don't forget to include bridge and highway tolls. Tolls may be deducted in addition to the mileage deduction.

Charitable contributions. The IRS might question whether or not a contribution reflects a business or a personal gift. Standard $10 and $25 donations to the well-known charities from the business are acceptable. A medical practitioner as a prominent member of the community is expected to support charities, especially the local ones. Five thousand dollars given to an obscure charity as a business gift rather than a personal one would be questioned. The deduction from the business rather than personal income results in a lower tax because of the way the self-employment tax is figured.

Filing systems

File all paid bills by vendor. Paid bills should be marked with the date of payment and the check number, or "paid in cash." Cancelled checks alone may not be sufficient to prove expenses. For example, a cancelled check to Ace Medical Supplies for $100 does not prove what was purchased. Paid bills constitute additional documentation of your expenses. Your cancelled checks, disbursement sheets (the ledger), and paid bills secure your audit trail. File the vendor cards separately. This set of records is kept more for convenience and for purposes of comparing expenses than for audit purposes. You may want to know how much a specific company charged for an item or how many items you need over a period of time. The cards also allow you to ascertain whether or not you have paid a particular vendor.

Petty cash

Careful record-keeping extends to your petty cash system. It is subject to abuse if it is kept in a sloppy fashion. And you won't be comfortable taking legitimate expense deductions if you don't have proper documentation. For example, you will find yourself paying for office supplies, miscellaneous photocopying, entertainment, postage, auto expenses, and small donations out of the petty cash box. These are all legitimate expenses and you will want a record of them.

There is a one-write system for petty cash to simplify the record-keeping. It consists of a ledger and voucher slips. Start with $100 in cash. Then everything should always add up to one hundred: the voucher slips plus the cash on hand and/or the ledger total plus the cash. Record the number of the slip, the name of the company or person paid, the date, and the amount in the appropriate ledger column (see Figure 7-2). Staple the receipt to the voucher slip and the transaction is complete. MasterCard can also be put through petty cash. Attach the receipt to the voucher. It is good for your staff to be disciplined in handling cash and to realize that you are not casual in this respect.

FEDERAL TAXES

Just as you no doubt consider it unwise for people to diagnose and treat a serious illness of their own, so it is unwise for medical practitioners earning, let's say, more than $10,000 to prepare their own income tax returns. However, rather than submit your financial affairs totally to another, it behooves you to be knowledgeable in tax matters, if only to be able to assist your accountant. Here we can do scarcely more than point out the obvious.

The form under which you conduct your practice will determine the way in which you will pay your taxes. If, for example, your business is a corporation, the corporation pays its own taxes on net income Form 1120. You will be an employee and, as such, will file a Form 1040 and pay a personal income tax. The corporation will withhold your income and social security tax from your salary, paying these taxes to the IRS quarterly.

However, if your business is in the form of the sole proprietorship, the procedure is somewhat different. There will be only one return—your own 1040. Rather than withholding, you will pay an estimated tax on Form 1040 ES each quarter that includes your income tax and social security tax. When people pay their own social security, the tax is called the Self-Employment Tax. Your personal return, the 1040, will include Schedule C, Profit (or Loss) from Business or Profession (Sole Proprietorship). On Schedule C you will report your

FIGURE 7-2
Cash control (petty cash)

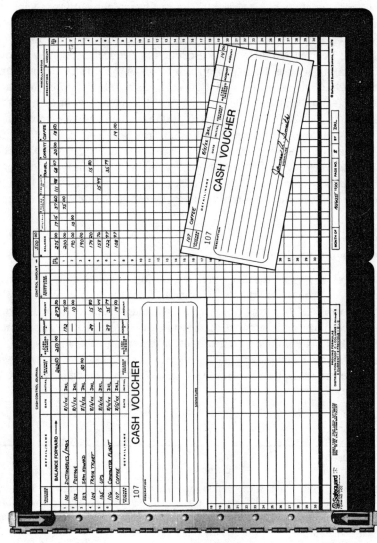

Form reprinted with permission from Safeguard Business Systems, 400 Maryland Drive, Fort Washington, Pennsylvania 19034.

gross income and expenses from your practice. The net profit or loss will be entered on your 1040.

The self-employment tax

If you work for no one but yourself, your self-employment tax (social security) will be based on the net income of your practice. But suppose you practice three days a week at a clinic. The clinic will not only withhold a portion of your salary for the IRS but will also make a deduction for social security, officially called Federal Insurance Contributions Act (FICA). In 1982 the maximum amount on which social security is figured is $32,400. Suppose you earned $25,000 at the clinic and had a net income of $10,000 from your own practice. You would subtract $25,000 from the $32,400 maximum and be responsible for paying a self-employment tax on only $7,400. You will have reached the maximum, so the difference between $7,400 and $10,000, i.e., $2,600, will not figure into the calculation of your self-employment tax. Similarly, if you change jobs and your new employer deducts FICA taxes as if none had yet been paid for that year, you can file for a return of any taxes figured on an amount above $32,400.

Paying taxes for employees

The federal government makes you responsible for collecting the taxes of your employees. You will withhold income tax from the salaries you pay, filing the proper form (4219) with the IRS quarterly and making regular deposits to the bank according to the amount of the sum owed. The FICA is paid at the same time. You, as employer, contribute to each employee's FICA. You must also pay a Federal Unemployment Tax on the first $6,000 of each employee's salary. At the end of the year you must give a receipt to each employee, the W-2

FIGURE 7-3
Federal taxes

Sole proprietorship	Corporation	Employers
Practitioner must file:	Corporation must file:	Employers must file:
1. Form 1040 plus	1. Form 1120.	1. Form 941 Employer's Quarterly Federal Tax Return. This includes withheld tax and FICA. Employer is liable for both the employee's share and the employer's share.
a. Schedule C Profit (and Loss) from a business.	2. Withholding, FICA, and unemployment tax for its employees.	
b. Self-employment tax schedule SE (1040).		
2. Must pay estimated tax quarterly (1040-ES).		2. Form 940 Federal Unemployment (FUTA).

form, showing the total amount withheld for the year and the total of FICA taxes paid.

Figure 7–3 outlines federal tax forms as discussed in this section.

What are your chances of an audit?

By means of a computer program the IRS picks up returns that are in some way unusual or contain serious errors, for example, a much higher or lower deduction than the average at a given income level. We have already mentioned a charitable donation of $5,000. It is the ratio of the amount to the gross that becomes conspicuous. This is not to say that you should not give away $5,000 if you want to, but show the deduction on your personal return and have documentation for it. You may also be audited because your return was among those randomly selected by another IRS computer program.

On page 163 of Publication 334 (revised November 1981) the IRS states:

> An examination of a taxpayer's return does not suggest a suspicion of dishonesty or criminal liability. It may not even result in more tax. Many cases are closed without change in reported tax liability and in many others the taxpayer receives a refund.

Notification of an audit comes in a polite computer-printed letter that describes audit procedure and requests certain records. "Tax returns are usually examined," according to the IRS, "to verify the correctness of income, exemptions, or deductions reported." You may bring an accountant, an attorney, or the person who prepared and signed your return. You do not have to be present.

Be prepared to defend items which are questioned. If you discover that you have inadequate documentation, negotiation is still possible if the examining agent feels that a compromise will expedite the audit. However, let your accountant defend his/her figures.

It is generally accepted that once the IRS succeeds in an audit, the chances are good that they will reaudit in the future, although there is no official IRS policy in this regard. Therefore, some perserverance in defending your claim is warranted. If a blatant error is caught by the IRS, it is best to take the consequences and pay back-taxes, fines, and interest. Interest, by the way, is calculated from the required date of filing to the date of the settlement. Although only about 2 or 3 percent of returns are audited, an audit is always a possibility. If you keep adequate records, leaving a well-documented audit trail, you should have no difficulty in proving your claims for legitimate deductible items.

LEGAL STRUCTURES

The legal structure you choose for your practice will determine the financial liability to which you will be subject as well as the form in which you will pay federal and state taxes and the ways in which you can raise capital. There are three legal structures which a practice as a business can adopt: a sole proprietorship, a partnership, and a corporation. Each legal structure differs in respect to legal, tax, and financial considerations.

Sole proprietorship

The simplest and cheapest form of organization is the sole proprietorship. A sole proprietorship is an unincorporated business, owned and operated by one person. It does not exist apart from you, the owner. Its liabilities are your liabilities. It is not necessary to file any legal forms to open a practice as a sole proprietor unless you plan to use a name other than your own. If you plan to call your practice *Modern Dentistry,* for example, you will probably have to file a trade name certificate with the town or city clerk. And when you open a bank account, you will probably be asked to show the certificate to the bank officer. Other than your state license to practice, no legal arrangements are necessary.

Sole proprietorship is a classification of the Internal Revenue Service. As such you will be required to keep financial records so that you can file a Schedule C of Form 1040. Schedule C is a statement of profit and loss for the business. As a part of your personal income tax return, you will show on Schedule C the costs of doing business, including the use of your home as an office, if such is the case. Your income is considered a draw and no member of your family including yourself may receive a salary.

Advantages and disadvantages. The principal disadvantage of sole proprietorship is legal liability. As a sole proprietor you are legally responsible for all debts and other obligations incurred by your business. That is, there is an unlimited liability. This liability extends to all the proprietor's assets, such as house and car. Personal assets can be protected by insurance but such insurance may be expensive. Professional liability can be covered by malpractice insurance. A second disadvantage is that illness or death of the proprietor would bring the business to a close. And third, a sole proprietor may be at a disadvantage in procuring long-term financing.

The major advantage of sole proprietorship is that the practice as a business is your own which you can operate as you see fit and the profits are all yours. Furthermore, there is a minimum of paper work, legal standards, and start-up costs. And finally there is a relative freedom from government control and special taxation. A practice can always start out as a sole proprietorship, and if there is a need, can be turned into a partnership or a corporation.

Partnership

A partnership is an association of two or more persons to carry on as co-owners of a business for profit. The participating partners normally put into writing in a partnership agreement the contributions of each partner and generally a delineation of the roles of the partners in the business relationship. Included also in the agreement would be a specification of the duration of the agreement, how business expenses will be handled, the individual authority of the partners in handling business matters, the division of profits and losses, draws and salaries, and settlement of disputes and arbitration. Of particular importance in a partnership agreement is the handling of the interests of a partner who dies as well as a process for the sale of a partnership interest.

Advantages of a partnership include the ease of formation (although a lawyer's help should be solicited in drawing up a partnership agreement), a greater ability to obtain capital, and a better range of skills among partners than in a sole proprietorship. Partnerships are not subject to any particular government controls or special taxation as are corporations.

Among the disadvantages of partnerships are unlimited liability on the part of at least one partner, an unstable life since elimination of one partner constitutes an automatic dissolution of the partnership (although there are legal means for continuing the business), and the difficulty of disposing of a partnership interest if not specifically arranged for in the partnership agreement.

A partnership is not a taxable entity but it must file a return for informational purposes with the Internal Revenue Service showing profit and loss. Each partner pays a tax or deducts the loss as a part of his or her own personal income tax.

Corporation

The corporation is by far the most complex of the three business structures. What sets it apart from the other two is its existence as an entity unto itself, distinct from the individuals who own it. It is a legal creation formed by the authority of a state government to conduct business as if it were an individual. As such, a corporation must file an income tax return and pay a corporate tax on profits. Individual shareholders also must pay a tax on the dividends they receive as shareholders. Thus, corporate profits are taxed twice. Associations of professional people organized under state professional association acts are generally recognized as corporations for federal income tax purposes.

A corporation is usually formed under the laws of the state where the corporation will conduct its business, although there may be tax (and other) advantages to incorporating in another state. Generally, the first step is the preparation of a certificate of incorporation. Many states have a standard certificate of incorporation which may be used by small business people. The following information will be requested: (1) the name of the corporation which must not resemble the name of any other corporation in the state; (2) the purposes for which the corporation is to be formed; (3) the length of time of its existence; (4) names and addresses of incorporators, amount and type of capital stock; (5) provisions for the regulation of internal affairs; and (6) provisions to amend the certificate of incorporation. If all is correct and proper, the certificate will be issued.

This is followed by a meeting of the stockholders to complete the incorporation process at which officers of the corporation are elected and by-laws adopted.

The disadvantages of the corporation as a legal structure lie in the burden of government regulation at the local, state, and federal level, including the number of reports that must be filed. For a very small business, such as a beginning health practice, the cost of forming a corporation might loom large. The double tax, mentioned above, is another important consideration.

Advantages of the corporation lie to a great extent in the limiting of liability to a fixed amount of investment, although no corporation will spare a doctor from personal liability in a malpractice suit. In addition, the ownership of the business is readily transferable through sale of stock and the corporation is relatively permanent. Another major consideration for those who need a large capital outlay is that the corporation may make it easier to raise money through the sale of stock. It may also be easier to secure long-term financing from lending institutions. The corporation also has the advantage of drawing on the skills of more than one person.

However, the chief advantage of the corporate structure for health professionals is that larger sums of money can be protected from income taxes for retirement purposes. The maximum limit that a sole proprietor can shelter from taxes is $7,500. Under the corporate structure practitioners can shelter from taxes an amount about equal to 25 percent of their salaries up to a limit of more than $40,000—a limit that is readjusted upward each year for inflation. For a fuller discussion of financial planning for retirement see Chapter 9.

Which structure is best for your business?

If you plan to conduct a small private practice while continuing to work for someone else, you will probably want to keep your affairs simple. By working out your own income tax for the first few years, perhaps under the guidance of your accountant, you will get a grasp of the issues as well as the vocabulary of accounting and taxes. When, and if, you decide to form a business with others, you will need to explore the legal and tax advantages of a partnership versus a corporation. Consult with your lawyer who should be able to outline for you the particular advantages and disadvantages for your practice.

As your affairs become more complicated, for example, you join forces with several other professionals for the sole purpose to buy or build an office building, you may want to review again some of the advantages and disadvantages of the corporate structure. When your practice becomes so successful that you have more than $7,500 to invest, you will surely want to investigate the tax incentive for retirement offered under the corporate structure. See the Annotated Bibliography for recommended reading.

8

Clinical records and other professional responsibilities

CLINICAL RECORDS

Good clinical records lie at the heart of any medical practice as a fundamental method of leaving behind a trail of evidence for each intervention in a patient's physical or mental state. First and foremost, clinical records maintain accountability to patients as well as to licensing and ethical boards. As a scientist, the practitioner will keep good records to evaluate diagnosis and treatment. Your training, too, has taught the value of careful and complete clinical records.

Above and beyond the call of ethics, professionalism, and science, there are the practical reasons for vigilance concerning clinical records—threats and promises to reward or punish you for your record-keeping. Good records will help you to get your bills paid. Insurance companies and government agencies, the third-party payers, require specific information based on your clinical record concerning a patient before they will OK a payment. Or you may become embroiled in a malpractice suit or a claim of unethical practice. Your records will constitute important evidence that shows your professional behavior was appropriate. In a court case, the evidence for innocence or guilt may depend on your records. And, of course, you will need to consult your records in any communication you have with other health professionals concerning a particular patient.

More important than any of these considerations is the need for you to know exactly what you saw, heard, and felt when you examined a patient—your diagnosis, your treatment plan, and any other information bearing on the health of a patient. The record provides a chronology of care, thought, and intervention for that patient. Thus, the record provides the practitioner with a continuity for a patient of what has been done and what is to be done. In written form, it defies deterioration of long- and short-term memory. And finally, keeping good records is a part of what you are being paid for.

The two requisites of good clinical records are:

1. Accuracy and completeness of factual information.
2. A retrieval system that gives ready access to that information.

These two requisites are in a sense contradictory. That is, the more complete and detailed the record is, the more difficult it may be to find any particular detail. For example, the psychiatrist who keeps a record of everything said by a client and self would soon find endless and useless volumes of material on file. The solution is to develop a system buttressed by innovative forms and procedures.

Medical histories

Medical histories have seven basic components: patient identification, chief complaint, history of present illness, past medical history, biographical data, family history, and a review of systems.

Patient identification. In many medical offices new patients are asked to complete a personal data card asking for such information as name, address, home and business phone numbers, insurance identification numbers, a person to call in case of an emergency, and the name and address of the person who will pay the bill if different from the patient. This is the information needed to prepare a patient ledger card for billing purposes (see Chapter 6, Income). The information should be kept up-to-date. The identification card is often stapled to the outside of the patient's file.

Chief complaint. Usually the chief complaint, the reason for the patient's request for care, is recorded in the patient's own words and so indicated by quotation marks. A record of the patient's perceived needs in a short and simple statement keeps in focus the patient's priorities for health care.

History of present illness. In recording the history of the present illness, and indeed the entire medical history, it is important that the record be factual, concise, and unbiased. There should be no interpretations of patient's behavior or personal comments. This is a record that may be read by the patient, by other professionals, by lawyers. The following are some suggestions for data to be elicited:

I. Introduction.
- A. Client's summary.
- B. Usual health.

II. Investigation of symptoms: chronological story.
- A. Onset.
- B. Date.
- C. Manner (gradual or sudden).
- D. Duration.
- E. Precipitating factors.
- F. Course since onset.
  1. Incidence (frequency).
  2. Manner.
  3. Duration (longest, shortest, and average times).
  4. Patterns of remissions and exacerbations.
- G. Location.
- H. Quality.
- I. Quantity.
- J. Setting.
- K. Associated phenomena.
- L. Alleviating or aggravating factors.

III. Negative information.

IV. Relevant family information.

V. Disability assessment.

(Malasanos et al., 1981)

Past history. The purpose of the past history is to place the present history in the context of the patient's life. The following are suggested areas for inquiry:

A. Past illnesses.
 1. Childhood illnesses.
 2. Injuries.
 3. Hospitalizations.
 4. Operations.
 5. Other major illnesses.
B Allergies.
 1. Environmental.
 2. Ingestion.
 3. Drug.
 4. Other.
C. Immunizations.
D. Habits.
 1. Alcohol.
 2. Tobacco.
 3. Drugs.
 4. Coffee, tea.
E. Medications taken regularly.
 1. By practitioner's prescription.
 2. By self-prescription.

(Malasanos et al., 1981)

Biographical data. Each practitioner will be interested in different aspects of a patient's life and will probably have worked out not only an interviewing style but a basic sequence in which questions are asked. The following are suggestions for eliciting biographical data that may have a bearing on a person's health:

 1. Sex.
 2. Occupation (present and usual).
 3. Diet.
 4. Sleep patterns.
 5. Military history.
 6. Hobbies, interests.
 7. Marital history.
 8. Children.
 9. Home life.
10. Religious conviction.
11. Race.
12. Social Security number.

13. Birthplace.
14. Source of referral.

(Adapted from Raus and Raus, 1974)

Family history. Many health problems are known to run in families either because of genetic or environmental factors. The following information is solicited aboout the mother, father, sisters, and brothers of the patient: age and health status, or age at death and cause, family diseases, serious illnesses, deformities, and allergies.

Review of systems. In this section each practitioner will conduct a line of questioning and a physical exam of the systems involved in his or her own specialty. A checklist should be routinely followed so that nothing is forgotten.

Formats

Most practitioners will want to chart a medical history on a form. A form systematizes the information with similar data always in the same place on the form. (Several forms are shown in Appendix III.) Some practitioners may want to work out a form for their own use. Asking other practitioners in a similar specialty about their forms will no doubt prove helpful.

The ongoing record

Every communication with, or about, a patient must be recorded and placed with the patient's ongoing record. This includes visits, examinations, telephone conversations, orders for lab tests, test results, release and consent forms, and particularly a continuing chronology of diagnoses, treatment, and progress. The result should be systematic and consistent from patient to patient. A diagnosis, for example, should be easy to find so that someone billing an insurance company can do so without assistance. Similarly, treatment, medication, and other such information should be logged in a consistent fashion.

One system (Ziegler, 1979) for keeping patient's medical records in useful order is seen in Figure 8–1.

1. Patient's history is summarized at the top of page.
2. A summary of problems and diagnoses is noted, one numbered line for each contact, and dated on the lower left side of same page.
3. On lower right is a line-by-line dated record of medications for each contact, according to number.

When the lines for problems and diagnoses, and medications are filled, a new blank form is stapled to the lower half of the page. Such a record forms a quick summary of a practitioner's experience with a patient with the chronolog-

FIGURE 8-1
Patient medical record

Name				Date of Birth		Date 1st Visit	File #

Family Hx

ROS

Social Hx

Allergies (D/?)

			PROBLEMS/DIAGNOSIS			MEDICATIONS	
No.	C/A	Date Entered	Item	Date Resolved	Date Entered	Item/Dosage	

From *Patient Records Control* by A. B. Ziegler, copyright © 1979 Litton Industries, Inc. Published by Medical Economics Company, Oradell, NJ 07649. All rights reserved.

ical record of problem, diagnosis, and medication set out in a clear and accessible fashion. Phone calls can be noted as well as lab results.

The detailed notes for each contact can be kept on a full sheet of paper and placed in the folder. Control over the record of each contact is maintained by numbering and dating the contact. If notes are made on a tape recorder to be typed later by a stenographer, they should be reviewed and initialed by the practitioner before becoming a part of the permanent record.

Patient files

Most practitioners keep patient records in pendaflex folders filed either alphabetically, or for a large or group practice, according to a numerical code in filing cabinets. Stapled to the outside of the folder will be the patient's identification card. Inside, the summary of the chronological record will lie on top of the remaining bulk of the material. Patient data should be kept in a consistent order. A copy of all correspondence pertaining to a patient should find its way into this record. Such items as correspondence, lab tests, and chronological notes should be kept in dated order with the most recent item on top.

Retaining records

How long must you keep clinical records? In New York State, for example, the law is specific. All patient records must be retained for at least six years. Obstetrical records and records of minor patients must be retained for at least six years and until one year after the minor patient reaches the age of 21 years. Consult a lawyer as to the legal length of time in your state. In addition, you should make some written provision or instruction for the disposal or transfer of patient records in the event of your own death.

You will not want to clutter your office with a collection of lifetime records but to keep your active patient files separate from the inactive ones. You might want to consider the following system with three sets of files: a current active file for patients currently being seen; a current inactive file for patients who come from time to time; and a storage file for patients you no longer see. This system entails a systematic combing out of the files at regular intervals.

1. *Current active files* would include charts of patients seen during the last three months—both patients with acute problems and those with chronic problems seen at regular intervals of less than three months time. There would be a monthly culling of patient charts to remove those of patients not seen within the past three months. The advantage is that the file is kept small enough to be convenient for daily usage. As current active patients call or lab reports come in, the file is ready at hand.

2. *Current inactive files* include charts of patients not seen within the last three months who *have* been seen within the last five years. These files should

be culled on a regular basis also, perhaps monthly or quarterly with charts older than five years placed in storage files.

3. *Storage files* should be kept as long as legally necessary. Some patient charts may be retained indefinitely for certain purposes. Keeping the files of some patients whom you have not seen for many years is an obligation, part of your responsibility to your patients. Many illnesses develop over a long period of time. Veterans, for example, have suffered complications 10 to 15 years or more after having been exposed to dangerous chemicals in the field. Their medical records have become important aspects in differential diagnoses.

Charts kept in numerical order are more easily culled than those alphabetized. Since numbers are assigned to patients chronologically, the charts can be checked by number without any further identification.

Appointment book

The appointment book is a permanent record in the same sense as a medical history or medical chart. It is not only a tool to keep track of the day's activity, it is a record of the services offered on a day-to-day basis and, as such, might constitute evidence in court or to the Internal Revenue Service. Practitioners who work in multiple locations usually have a master book to coordinate activities. A small book that you carry around with you for appointments is a useful tool. If a receptionist also makes appointments for you, have your book updated on a regular basis. Your appointment book also serves as a backup to your daily log of accounts receivable. You can use it for a quick check on cancellations and fee collections.

CONFIDENTIALITY

Health practitioners must be sensitive to the fact that an illness, even a visit to a doctor, can constitute incriminating evidence against a patient. Facts about the health of individuals is private and privileged information. No matter how humdrum any particular item might be, even as innocent a matter as a person's height and weight, it is nonetheless, nobody else's business. The confidentiality of patients' medical records cannot be overemphasized both to health practitioners and to the administrative personnel who maintain their records.

Furthermore, it is illegal to allow access to clinical records without the express permission of the individual to whom the records pertain according to the Privacy Act of 1974. Only in cases in which a third party has the legal authority to do so or when public health considerations supersede a patient's right to privacy, can a client's right to privacy be breached.

There are numerous occasions when a practitioner is asked for information concerning a patient. Insurance companies, law enforcement agencies, schools, potential employers, and others—all may ask for clinical information concerning a patient. Insurance companies sometimes provide a blanket release as a part of a standard form. Such releases may be too broad or too old to be considered valid for releasing information. Oftentimes patients sign releases without any idea of what they are to be used for. Although you cannot deny access to records if a patient has unwittingly signed a release, you can set certain standards. Authorizations to release information should be recent and signed. Some rules concerning such authorizations might be as follows:

1. A release form must specify the person or agency to whom the disclosure is to be made.
2. The purpose of the disclosure must be specified.
3. The release must have been signed within 30 days with a handwritten date or within six months if notarized.
4. Do not release information over the phone with or without a patient's authorization. However, if the request is from another health care professional, you can verify that person's identity by calling back to provide the requested information.
5. When forwarding information by mail, do not send the entire record. Only the pertinent information is necessary.
6. If the entire medical record is requested, you may send a face sheet, a summary of the present situation, and the patient's history (DeWitt, 1981).

When patients want to see their records

Until the rise of the right to privacy issue and the enactment of laws protecting personal records, there was a situation in which "there [was] somewhat casual access to the record by almost everyone *except* the patient (DeWitt, 1981). As of early 1981, 24 states had enacted laws giving people the right to see their records.[1] According to one lawyer, "The medical record is owned by the [health professional] and is the property of the [health professional] . . . but in the great majority of states the [health professional] may not hold the record in such a way as to prevent patient access to it" (Friedman, 1981).

Since patient records are essentially kept and organized for the practitioner's professional purposes and not in a form readily accessible to the layman, health care practitioners must establish a policy regarding this issue. One suggestion concerns the content of the record. Bear in mind while you are taking your notes that at some time the patient may want to see them. Keep your notes factual. Write only what you actually see and hear, what your intervention consists of, what drugs, and so forth. Avoid any gratuitous personal judgments.

Patients can arrive at a misconception about themselves after reading a clinical record unassisted; even patients who may seem to be quite knowledgeable

---

[1]The states in question are Alaska, California, Colorado, Connecticut, Florida, Illinois, Indiana, Louisiana, Maine, Maryland, Massachusetts, Michigan, Minnesota, Mississippi, Montana, Nevada, New York, Oklahoma, Oregon, Rhode Island, South Dakota, Tennessee, Virginia, and Wisconsin.

about the health field. One such patient, a man who had a friend who had recently died of leukemia, saw from his record that he had what seemed like a tremendous number of white blood cells and erroneously jumped to the conclusion that he too had leukemia. Therefore, when you comply with such requests, you will want to be considerate of the patient as well as to protect yourself and the records. The following suggestions might be helpful:

1. Review the record yourself before showing it to a patient to be sure it is complete and in proper order. There is always the chance that something has been slipped into a folder that doesn't belong there.
2. Do not leave the person alone with the record. He or she might alter it or remove something from the folder.
3. Do not allow any material to be removed from your office.
4. Patients have a right to a copy of their records. If you have a copier, you can charge a minimum fee per page or you can have copies made outside.
5. The best arrangement is to actually read the record to the patient so that you can explain not only the terminology and the abbreviations, but the meaning and prognosis of the person's illness.

What about minors? Parents have to be given access to the records of their minor children. This is a particularly thorny question for mental health practitioners, gynecologists, and even pediatricians. Reporting children's confidences as well as their activities to their parents will scarcely encourage the trust of young patients. One psychiatrist who specializes in adolescents tells parents that he will tell them if something is life-threatening thus discouraging unnecessary parent inquiries. The way in which confidences will be handled should be discussed with parents and children the first time the child is seen.

Emergencies

The most dramatic example of the release of information without specific permission might be an emergency situation in which a patient calls a psychotherapist to say that he or she is about to commit suicide. The patient is alone and lives 10 miles away. A sensible response on the part of the mental health practitioner would have to be to forget about confidentiality and call the police. Similarly, if a patient says that he or she is going to kill someone, warnings must be given. However, you need only reveal that amount of information about your patient which is critical to the immediate situation.

MALPRACTICE

A malpractice claim or even the threat of one can be exceedingly stressful and harmful to a private practitioner. There is not only the possibility of a large sum of money being awarded to the patient and serious injury to the practitioner's reputation, but a malpractice claim can cause a practitioner a great deal of time and personal anguish. For protection and aid in case of a claim being brought against you as well as peace of mind, it is advisable to carry malpractice insurance. However, excessive fear of malpractice claims is unrealistic according to the evidence of various surveys and other studies of malpractice claims brought against hospitals and private practitioners. There are also lessons to be learned from these studies about patients' perceptions and expectations of the health professions in examinations of the reasons patients bring malpractice claims.

Statistics from the surveys

Although the statistics on the incidence of malpractice claims show a wide variation, there is general agreement that there has been an alarming increase in claims in the last 20 years. This is reflected in significant increases in insurance rates. During the 1960s, for example, the average premiums paid by surgeons rose 950 percent and even those for dentists more than doubled (Curran, 1979). Data indicate that the number of malpractice claims increased 20 percent each year from 1970 to 1976 (Fifer, 1979). However, malpractice claims don't just fall like the rains from heaven equally on all. Of all loss dollars paid by insurance companies from July 1975 to June 1976, 85 percent were for claims originating in hospital settings and 81 percent relate to surgery or postsurgical care. (See Tables 8–1 and 8–2.) The same study found that 70 percent of the claims paid were against surgeons, particularly orthopedists, obstetricians/

TABLE 8–1
Twelve leading allegations in malpractice claims*

Allegations	Number of claims	Percent
Improper treatment		
Surgical error	1,747	20
Lack of supervision, control	809	10
Fracture or dislocation	712	8
Birth-related problems	648	7
Surgical, postoperative	623	7
Surgical, improper procedure	607	7
Drug side effect	579	7
Infection	554	6
Failure to diagnose		
Fracture or dislocation	803	9
Cancer	552	6
Surgery		
Postoperative complication	650	7
Lack of informed consent	442	5
Total	8,726	

*Based on an analysis of claims against the St. Paul Company for October through December 1977.

W. R. Fifer, "Risk Management and Medical Malpractice," *Quality Review Bulletin*, April 1979.

TABLE 8-2
Principal procedures involved in production of class I potentially compensable events*

Procedure	Number of PCEs†	Procedure	Number of PCEs
Hysterectomy, total	43	Hip arthroplasty	14
Radiation therapy	36	Heart valve procedures	13
Term delivery	27	Repair of abdominal	
Fractured hip, open		aneurysms	12
reduction	23	Cataract extraction	11
Cholecystectomy	22	Appendectomy	10
Colectomy, partial	21	Other fractures, open	
Transurethral resection		reduction	10
of prostate	20	Pacemaker insertion	10
Gastrectomy, partial	19	Hiatal hernia, abdominal	
Exploratory laparatomy	18	approach	8
Tonsillectomy/		Inguinal hernia	8
adenoidectomy	18	Craniotomy	6
Intravenous discectomy	16	Hemorrhoidectomy	5
Cesarean section	15	Middle ear procedures	5

*These data were derived from the California Medical Insurance Feasibility Study (CMIFS).
W. R. Fifer, "Risk Management and Medical Malpractice," *Quality Review Bulletin*, April 1979.

gynecologists, plastic surgeons, head and neck surgeons, and neurosurgeons (AMA, 1978, in Fifer, 1979). The typical defendant in a malpractice action has been characterized as a board-certified physician in the prime of life (Richards, 1978). However, in another study of physicians in Los Angeles it was shown that there was a concentration of suits brought against a very small group of physicians (46 of 8,000) who accounted for 10 percent of all claims and 30 percent of all payments made in a four-year period (Schwartz and Komisar, 1978, in Fifer, 1979).

The number of suits brought to a successful conclusion for the claimant is surprisingly small as are the dollar amounts awarded. For example, in one study it was shown that 90 percent of the claims brought were settled out of court and of those that did go to trial, 80 percent were won by the defendant physician or hospital (Curran, 1979). The median award was $2,000 and only 3 percent were over $100,000. In 1970, of 382,000 doctors, dentists, and hospitals with malpractice insurance, one out of every 21 were sued (Curran, 1973).

Why do patients sue?

Despite protests by health professionals that many malpractice suits are "frivolous" in nature (Vaccarino, 1977), there is evidence that the number of malpractice claims are only the tip of the iceberg (only one in six malpractice incidents result in a claim) and those claims are rooted in medical injury and malpractice (Somers, 1977; Brook and Williams, 1978). The evidence shows that patients sue because harm has been done and negligence can be demonstrated.

A question more helpful to the practitioner might be, why is it that only one in six patients who had cause, actually sued. In other words, is there something to be done that can prevent suits in addition to giving high quality care? The answer seems to lie in the patient/practitioner relationship. A rapport between practitioner and patient can help patients to anticipate the experience that lies ahead in solving their health problems. When the outcome is not as expected and the private practitioner gives only cursory attention or the patient feels he or she has been poorly provided for, a suit "is often the tangible proof of the final breakdown of [that] human relationship" (HEW, 1973). If, on the other hand, patients feel that their welfare matters to their private practitioners, that they are doing all in their power to help, then it is unlikely a malpractice suit will be filed, regardless of the outcome.

The principal direct cause of malpractice claims is a poor result—any outcome that fails to meet the expectation of a patient. Sometimes such situations are set up because so many people have misconceptions as to what modern medicine actually can do. In addition to communicating your concern to a patient, you must also view yourself as a teacher or explainer. You may perform a certain procedure 10 times in the course of a week, but to each patient it is probably a new experience. Take the time to explain before and after an operation or any other procedure and to answer any questions. Explanations of what can realistically be accomplished and of the risks associated with the various choices of treatments will help to avoid the bitter disappointments that can lead to a malpractice claim. A well thought out disclosure for faciomaxial surgery is included in Appendix V. Involving patients and their families in some of the decision making helps them to understand that medical practice does not necessarily provide clear-cut directions, that each case is a little different, and that medical practitioners can only use their best judgment based on their knowledge, skill, and experience.

When patients have questions about results, they need extra attention immediately. According to one expert (Vaccarino, 1977), this is the most crucial phase of the claims sequence. What is done by the practitioner when a patient is disappointed in an outcome, may either stop a potential claim or force a patient to see a lawyer. If you are arrogant, distant, not available often enough, or difficult to talk to, then the patient may begin to question clinical competence. Remember that patients are usually not qualified to judge your clinical competence. They can only judge you as they see you—based on your actions as a human being. Your clinical competence alone, cannot protect you against a claim being brought against you.

A triggering cause of malpractice suits is often a staggering bill from the doctor and the hospital. The three in combination—a poor patient/practitioner relationship, an unexpected poor result, topped off by a demand for a large sum of money can produce the anger that leads a patient or a patient's family to the malpractice lawyer. Everyone is surely aware of the skyrocketing costs of modern medicine, but not always as it may apply to themselves and so can be dumb-founded by a medical bill. Often patients believe they are covered by insurance for all of the costs. This is not always true. A talk about money before the expense is incurred can soften the blow. The conversation should include an estimate of the bill and possible ways of meeting the payment. An insensitive billing process often acts as the irritant that results in a malpractice claim.

Legal definitions of negligence

The assumption that has been made in this discussion of malpractice claims is that health professionals are practicing at a high level of competence and that they are keeping up with the standard of care in their field. This is their legal obligation as well as an obligation to their patients. Professional liability suits in most cases involve allegations that the health practitioner "has diagnosed or treated a patient's illness 'negligently'" (Holder, 1973). Negligence is the legal term for omission of care in a situation in which another person has been in-jured by that omission on the part of the health professional. Legally the plain-tiff must prove that the standard of care rendered was not sufficient. As you can see, legally, negligence is defined according to the conception of "standard of care" in any particular case.

Standard of care is defined by the courts as (1) the degree of ability or skill possessed by other professionals in the same locality, (2) the degree of care and diligence ordinarily exercised by those professionals in their practice, and (3) the extraordinary skill or ability of a specialist, if the person involved claims a specialty. In other words, you are allowed to make mistakes. The law does not demand more than that which another professional in the same situation could have done. The standard is set according to the general standard of care and knowledge in the health community—"the ability possessed by the average member of the health profession in good standing." You will not incur liability for mistakes if the methods you used are recognized and approved by those reasonably skilled in your field (Holder, 1973).

Because the court has no way of knowing what the standard of care might be, health professionals are frequently in the courts giving expert testimony on diagnoses and treatments that conform to the standard of care in a particular case. That means that in a malpractice case your management of a patient will be judged by others in your field and your defense will be that you have treated your patient according to accepted practice. You need only prove that there are other professionals who would have performed similarly to the way you did. You can produce your own expert witness to testify that your diagnosis and treatment conforms to an acceptable standard of care.

What you can do to prevent malpractice claims

In the final analysis you cannot prevent a malpractice claim brought by a patient somehow outraged at the treatment he or she received. Everyone has the right to seek redress of an alleged wrong in the courts. However, there are many things you can do to prevent malpractice claims in the ordinary course of your practice. First, and foremost, is practicing to the best of your ability and keeping up with your field. That really goes without saying.

Rapport. We have spoken already of the importance of good rapport with patients. Rapport also means that you make yourself available when a patient is disturbed by the outcome of a procedure as well as explaining possible outcomes and the risks involved. A good patient relationship means that you must learn how to talk about money with patients and make yourself or someone on your staff an expert in health insurance so that you can explain to patients just what they can expect the insurance company or government agency to pay and about how much they must expect to pay themselves.

Medical records. Once a malpractice claim has been made against you, your principal defense will be your clinical records. Your records contain the documentation to prove that your standard of care conformed to acceptable standards. The record must speak for itself. It must be accurate, detailed, and unambiguous. If you departed from the usual practice, there should be a notation in the record that you did so and why you did so. You will be protected against what turned out to be a wrong diagnosis if the record shows that you exercised diligence in your reasoning.

> In the objective, interpretive, and plan sections of the progress notes, the professional has a chance to reveal exactly why he took a given course of action, exactly what he chose to neglect, exactly what his priorities were . . . and, most important, why he may have deviated from the usual criteria for the management of a specific problem (Weed, 1971; quoted by Vaccarino, 1977).

One good way to think about what the medical record should contain might be to think about what you would want to see if you were called in as a new consultant on the case in order to understand the history and to start a course of treatment. The record is not a personal diary and should, of course, contain no subjective comments and should be written in a professional style.

Communication. If you work in a hospital setting, it is recommended (Fifer, 1979; Rubin, 1978; Vaccarino, 1977) that you alert other staff members, particularly those who will come in contact with your patient, as well as appropriate members of the administration staff, that your patient has complaints and is a possible candidate for bringing a malpractice suit. A little attention and care on the part of the hospital staff may be able to head off the problem.

What to do if a claim of malpractice is brought against you

The lawyer is by training (and perhaps by disposition) contentious—an advocate and a taker of sides. People in the health professions, on the other hand, are trained as mediators. Their concerns are humanistic and they would like to be viewed as they view themselves—as people whose primary purpose is to help others. So that except perhaps for surgeons, who may be sued more than once in their professional careers and become more sophisticated about the process, private practitioners who are sued, are likely to be consumed with anxiety, guilt, remorse, or depression. In short, accused practitioners will probably find themselves in a crisis situation. In such a state of mind, they may take inappropriate actions.

The first thing to do is to recognize that a lawsuit is a competition—an adversarial situation with a winner and a loser and that the opposing side will try to take every advantage they can of the situation. You will probably make an immediate review of the case in question and begin a frantic process of soul searching and self-evaluation. Your immediate impulse may be to call the plaintiff—your patient—and try to use reason or even call the plaintiff's attorney. Such an attempt, if it works, would be brilliant, but the likelihood is that you will only further enrage the plaintiff and give him or her cause to accuse you of a coverup. Another pitfall is the desire to discuss the problem with a colleague or friend. Be aware that any written narrative of the events or discussions on the subject can be subjected to an examination of the minutest details in dispositions, interrogatories, or the courtroom itself by a hostile and challenging questioner. If you must talk to a colleague, present the case as a hypothetical situation and don't give anyone any written account of the situation. The more you regard yourself as innocent of the charges, the more self-righteous and indiscreet you may be (Wright, 1981).

So what do you do? You notify your carrier just as you would do if your house had been broken into. And then you wait. Try to keep in mind that the litigation process takes time and is one that profits by delay. If the uncertainty becomes too much for you, consult your personal attorney (your conversation will be privileged) or better yet, a private attorney knowledgeable about malpractice in your field. Such an attorney can educate you to the legal intricacies of malpractice cases and answer many of your questions.

The most important positive step you can take is to assemble all the documents and records that have any relevancy to the situation, such as, schedules, logs, case notes, reports, consent forms, notes from secretaries, colleagues, and notes detailing phone calls. The patient's records are the most important evidence in any liability suit, regardless of the factual issues involved (Holder, 1974).

A word of caution might be added here. Any alteration of the record will surely be construed as a "deliberate attempt to evade liability when negligence has occurred. And, in fact, may remove a case from the realms of civil suits and place it within the scope of criminal prosecution" (Holder, 1974). If it becomes necessary to alter or change the record, care should be taken not to raise any suspicion that the record has been "doctored" for ulterior purposes. Explanations should be noted for any changes made and dated at the time of the change.

A systematic chronicle of contacts with the patient will help you to remember what happened and will be invaluable to the defense lawyer. Do not show this material to anyone but your defense lawyer. You may also want to review the literature relevant to the type of case involved. You may find it reassuring and it will also be valuable in the formal defense (Wright, 1981).

A SURVIVOR'S CHECKLIST

Do

1. Recognize a personal crisis.
2. Promptly notify professional liability broker–carrier.
3. Consult personal attorney and/or seek referral to an experienced malpractice defense attorney.
4. Be patient. Recognize that the process of litigation may involve months and often years.
5. Begin a systematic and thorough review of the chronology and documentation of the case. Prepare a written summary to guide you. Organize all pertinent professional material (e.g., diagnostic protocols, case notes, memoranda, etc.). Show this to no one except when asked to do so by *your* attorney.
5a. Review the literature pertinent to the case.
6. If professional consultation regarding case management is desired, see a fellow practitioner only after consulting your attorney. If unable to consult your attorney, discuss the central issues of the case with your consultant/colleague only in hypothetical terms. Remember that professional case consultation is generally *not* considered privileged information.
7. Be especially thoughtful and discreet concerning the case in *all* communications with institutional representatives, institutional colleagues, practitioners from other disciplines, and so on. Remember that in most cases, there is an inherent conflict of interest between yourself as service provider and representatives, colleagues, and practitioners attached to involved institutions.
8. Maintain helpful and cooperative attitudes with the broker–carrier-retained attorney but periodically review strategy and *all* proposed settlements with your own attorney *before* irrevocably committing yourself.

Don't

1. Do not panic.
1a. Do not discuss the case injudiciously without legal safeguards such as privileged communication.
2. Do not attempt to settle matters yourself without proper legal guidance and/or without having worked through the matter personally.
3. Do not mail "virtuous" (or hostile or angry) letters to the client(s) involved.

4. Do not distribute *any* documents or similar material without prior clearance from your attorney.
5. Do not get trapped by a "friendly" attorney for the plaintiff(s) who "just wants to settle the unfortunate matter."
6. Do not get trapped into appearing to claim greater knowledge or expertise than can be objectively substantiated.

(Wright, 1981)

9

Financial protection

FINANCIAL PROTECTION

It is not possible to be protected completely from the indiscriminate blows that life hands out—from the fall in the bathtub to the fall of the national economy. However, there are a number of ways in which the prudent can arrange for a safety net in case of a disaster or even a slight misfortune. For those who are employed, the safety net usually is referred to as fringe benefits. Fringe benefits are an important part of the remunerative system and will include such features as health insurance, workman's compensation, disability insurance, unemployment insurance, pensions, and a discount on stock in the employing corporation. Self-employed private practitioners must, of course, take care of benefits and investments for themselves.

To what extent will private practitioners want to buy protection for themselves and their families? How much is enough and what kind of protection is the best dollar buy? The immediate answer depends on the age and family situation of the individual practitioner. For a man in his 30s with three young children and a wife who is totally occupied in bringing up the children and acting as a support system for her husband, the answer becomes "the works" or as much as the practitioner can afford. For a woman with no children and a husband who is financially successful and carries family health insurance, the answer might be just enough protection to keep her office going in case she is sick. However, she might wish to be financially independent of her husband and would seek full coverage for an early retirement and for her old age. In other words, the amount of financial protection one should provide for oneself and one's family becomes a matter of personal preference and of need. In general, the following kinds of protection can be purchased:

1. In case of sickness.
   a. The cost of medical care.
   b. Payments to compensate for loss of income.
   c. Payments to cover the cost of operating an office.
2. In case of death of the breadwinner or the homemaker.
   a. Life insurance.
3. Retirement and old age.
   a. Investments and savings.
   b. Tax-shelter plans, i.e., IRA and Keogh plans.

Health insurance

No health professional needs to be reminded of the astronomical cost of medical care nor of the fact that medical costs for the past few years have been among the leaders in the rate of increase. All the more reason for the health professional to purchase and maintain health insurance coverage. Since the collection problems involved in third-party payments provide the health professional with an extraordinarily detailed expertise on the various forms of health insurance and the coverage offered, we will not go into detail.

Health insurance, or rather, insurance in case of illness, comes in three different packages. Regardless of age or family circumstances (unless you are over 65 and eligible for Medicare), the health practitioner should purchase all three. The first is hospitalization and covers the cost of all or most of the hospital charges for a stay in a hospital. The second covers other basic medical expenses incurred in a hospital, particularly surgery, doctor's visits, diagnostic tests, etc. The third is usually called major medical and picks up where numbers one and two leave off.

Here are a few things to consider when buying your own health insurance.

Major medical. John Gregg, author of *The Health Insurance Racket and How to Beat It* (1973) advises that major medical coverage should receive first consideration in health insurance planning. What becomes financially unbearable is the case of a major disaster—a long term, expensive illness of any member of your family. So that when you examine the terms of an insurance policy you should be less interested in coverage from the first day, which you will be able to absorb, than long-term coverage for the catastrophe. When comparing major medical policies, examine not only the maximum limit of total payment but the internal limit, that is the maximum payments for each day in the hospital and for surgery and other medical costs.

Deductibles. A good principle to bear in mind when purchasing any kind of insurance is to try to absorb as much of the loss yourself by the use of deductibles. You will save money in the long run. With health insurance, and particularly major medical, the higher the deductible, that is the amount you will pay yourself before the insurance company picks up the bill, the lower the cost. Also, the longer the waiting period (the period of time from purchase of the policy to the availability of the benefits), the lower the cost (sometimes even 25 percent less).

Group. Buying health insurance as an individual is the costliest way to proceed. If you are employed part time, try to get in on a group plan. If that isn't possible, you may be able to form your own group if you employ one or more persons. Other group arrangements include membership in your professional organizations, fraternal associations, or alumni associations. If you are forced to leave an employee group when you establish your own practice, it is often possible to keep the group policy as an individual, perhaps at a higher cost or reduced coverage. However, a group policy may not provide all the coverage you need, particularly major medical.

The "Blues." If you are unable to buy health insurance as a member of a group, the next best buy is Blue Cross/Blue Shield. The Blues are universally recognized by hospitals so that at the very least you will be able to get in and out of a hospital with a Blues membership.

Private insurance companies offer not only more expensive coverage, but may prove difficult to deal with when it comes time for them to pay out. Buying health insurance by mail order or from salesmen who are not members of the community is a well-known hazard. Avoid them yourself and warn your patients against them.

What provisions should a health policy contain? It is of first importance that the policy be noncancellable and guaranteed renewable. That means that the company cannot cancel the policy at the end of the period. Such policies can be purchased up to the age of 50. There should be a provision calling for the nonpayment of premiums during a period of disability. Read the exclusions carefully. What physical conditions, illnesses, or accidents are excluded (not covered)? How much time must elapse before the actual coverage goes into effect? Remember, the longer you wait, the cheaper the coverage.

HMOs. Health Maintenance Organizations, in which health insurance is paid in advance to a group of doctors, may make a lot of sense for a young practitioner with a family. Perhaps practitioners feel they can avail themselves of professional courtesy, but over the long run, unless there is reciprocity between particular doctors, you may be more comfortable paying for regular health care for your family. If you belong to an HMO and have already paid for health care, you and the members of your family may be less reluctant to call the doctor in the case of an illness or an accident and more willing to schedule regular check-ups. Most prepayment plans include the cost of hospitalization which gives HMO members the opportunity to buy hospitalization at a substantially lower cost than private membership. Finally, as a health professional, you are in a good position to evaluate the competence of the participating doctors in the group.

Paying for your office when you are sick

The loss of income and the costs of medical care are not the only financial hardships suffered when a private practitioner becomes ill. Money must be spent to pay such fixed costs of doing business as salaries, rent, phone, etc., even when you are not there. Some professional groups offer such insurance at very low rates and, if you can buy such insurance for little money from your professional group, it may well be worthwhile.

LIFE INSURANCE

Over the many years that life insurance has been a major service industry, many gimmicks have been developed to sell life insurance. A principal one that works to confuse the issue is the selling of life insurance as an investment—the "so-it-shouldn't-be-a-total-loss" syndrome. At the outset it is important to distinguish between insurance and investment. An investment is a way to put your money to work for you to make more money. Insurance is a way to protect your family financially in the case of your death. In this section we will be talking about financial protection in the event of the death of the family breadwinner.

Do you need insurance?

Many people really have no need to buy life insurance. At best it may be a lottery for a beneficiary. At worst it is a way for an insurance salesperson to make a living. The key question is, are there people dependent upon your earning power for their livelihood? If not, you do not need life insurance. If you don't support anyone but yourself, don't buy any. If, on the other hand, you have a wife and several children or parents whom you support, you will want to provide for them in the case of your untimely death.

How much insurance should you buy?

Life insurance is costly as well as a fixed yearly expense. It is well worth your time to work out the amount of income your family will need and how much insurance you will need to insure that income. Relying on an insurance broker, no matter how good a friend, is not in your best interest. Insurance salespeople work on a commission basis and may recommend an insurance package that pays a better percentage for them rather than a policy that best protects your family. If you have small children the total amount you will need may be surprisingly high. With help of the worksheet (Figure 9-1) you can

FIGURE 9-1
How much insurance do you need?

WORKSHEET

Needs

A. Final expenses
  1. Funeral expenses $_____
  2. Probate costs   _____
  3. Medical expenses   _____
  4. Repayment of debt   _____
B. Long-term expenses
  1. Family living expenses $_____
  2. Emergency fund   _____
  3. Education fund   _____
  4. Retirement fund for spouse   _____
    Total expenses $_____

Assets
1. Social Security $_____
2. Current life insurance   _____
3. Pension benefits   _____
4. Cash and savings   _____
5. Equity in real estate   _____
6. Securities   _____
7. Other assets   _____

Total needs minus total assets equals additional insurance needed
Total needs $_____
Total assets   _____
Additional insurance needed $_____

calculate your needs, your assets, and the gap that must be filled by insurance. Your assumption is that you might die tomorrow. How much money will your survivors need immediately and in the long run?

Using the worksheet: Expenses

A. Final expenses.

1. Your survivors will have to pay your *funeral expenses* and the *legal costs of probating your will*. Although the state can distribute your assets, it is advisable to have a will. It may save you money and your lawyer can estimate for you the probate costs. In addition, you may have some uninsured *medical expenses* that will have to be met.

2. *Repayment of debts.* You will want to provide for payment of any debts you have incurred such as car payments, credit-card installment fund, and bank loans. Do you own your own home? Will it be sold and become an asset or will your family continue to live in it and have to make mortgage payments? You can buy mortgage insurance which will pay off the mortgage in case of your death, but Consumer Reports (1981) recommends that you include mortgage payments as a part of family expenses.

B. Long-term expenses.

1. *Family living expenses.* For the long term, family living expenses are the principal burden a life insurance plan must be prepared to carry. You can work out the figures from your family budget or figure on 75 percent of your after-taxes income.

2. *Emergency fund.* Include an extra lump sum to cover emergencies. Examples of an emergency might be the need of a new furnace or roof for the house or orthodontia for one of the children.

3. *Education fund.* The cost of a college education has skyrocketed in recent years. A degree from a private college can cost upwards of $50,000. With several children it is unrealistic to try to provide the complete amount plus, possibly, graduate school, but a sum to get them started or to cover much of a state or city school will give your children a good start. They will have to fend for themselves to some extent. They may have to anyway even if you are there to help them.

4. *Retirement funds for spouse.* Your spouse will receive Social Security benefits for herself and the children until the youngest child reaches the age of 18 or, if in school, 22. Your spouse will probably be in her middle 40s at that time. If she is not working now, her best insurance is to plan to work at that time and to prepare herself with some kind of training. Some kind of a retirement nest egg would be necessary from age of 65 until her own death to supplement the Social Security benefits she will receive. You may prefer to build up a retirement fund by means of investment rather than insurance for this purpose. For example, an annual deposit of $1,500 in an Individual Retirement Fund

(IRA), a government-sponsored tax shelter, at 8 percent will yield $45,740 in just 15 years.

Using the worksheet: Assets

1. *Social Security.* Social Security is the major protection that most Americans can count on in the case of the death of the breadwinner, but it will probably not take care of all of the needs of your family. If you are not sure of your eligibility, contact your local Social Security office. It is difficult to determine the exact amount your family would receive in the event of your death. If you have consistently earned the maximum Social Security-taxed wage, then use Tables 9–1 and 9–2 to figure the income of your survivors. Suppose you are 35

TABLE 9–1
Average Indexed Yearly Earnings (AIYE) based on maximum payments of Social Security tax each year

Age	AIYE
29 or less	$20,352
30	19,464
35	17,532
40	16,020
45	15,072
50	14,532
51–62	14,496

Social Security pays survivors' benefits based on the amount you have paid into the fund. There is a maximum on which you pay which has been increased in recent years. If you have paid that maximum each year, you can find your Average Indexed Yearly Earnings (AIYE) from the table, based on your age.
Source: *Consumer Reports*, February 1980.

with two children, the youngest age five, and both are in school until their 22nd birthday. The family will collect Social Security benefits for 17 years at the rate of about $860 a month. That comes to an overall figure of $174,440. So that, basically, the problem of deciding on how much insurance is needed is to provide for the gap between that figure and the total of all expenses.

With your AIYE go into Table 9–2 to determine survivor's benefits.

2. *Current life insurance.* You may have already purchased life insurance through a professional or fraternal association.

3. *Pension benefits.* You may already have opened an IRA or Keogh account. This money would become available to your family in the event of your death.

4. *Cash and savings.* Add up the total of savings and checking accounts and include here any Certificates of Deposit.

TABLE 9-2
Monthly Social Security survivors' benefits based on AIYE of wage earner

Your AIYE	Surviving parent and one child	Surviving parent and two children	One surviving child	Widow's or widower's benefit (starting at age 65)	Family maximum
$1,400	$183	$ 183	$122	$122	$ 183
$2,400	265	265	132	177	265
$4,800	361	361	180	241	361
$6,600	433	482	216	289	482
$8,400	505	613	252	337	613
$10,200	577	707	288	385	707
$12,000	649	771	324	433	771
$14,400	737	860	369	492	860
$16,200	771	900	386	514	900
$18,000	805	939	402	537	939
$20,400	850	992	425	567	992
$22,200	884	1,031	442	589	1,031
$22,900	897	1,046	448	598	1,046

Source: *Consumer Reports*, February 1980.

5. *Equity in real estate.* If you own your own home but the family plans to live there after your death, the value of your home can not be included. However, any other real estate that would be sold should be included, such as your office or rental income on a real estate investment.

6. *Securities.* You would include under this heading any corporate stocks and bonds, government bonds, or other investments.

7. *Other assets.* Include here any things you own that would be sold upon your death such as jewelry, collectibles, artwork, or an extra car. Be conservative in your estimates of the value of such items since values change and it is sometimes hard to realize the full purchase value of collectibles.

In the foregoing discussion the problem has been presented in terms of a family with a father who is the breadwinner and a mother and children who are dependents because it is the most common situation in which life insurance is needed. However, the woman health professional with small children should seriously consider the need the family would have for insurance in the case of her own death. The cost of replacing her income and her services might be very great indeed. The children might be eligible for Social Security survivors' benefits but if the surviving father earns more than $20,000 a year he would not be eligible.

What kind of insurance is the best buy

With minor wrinkes, there are basically two kinds of life insurance: (1) term and (2) cash value, sometimes called ordinary life.

Term insurance. As the name implies, term insurance covers the life of the insured only for a specific term, which might be anywhere from one to five years. After the term is up, when the insured buys the policy again, it will be at a higher rate because he or she is five years older. There is no cash accrual from the premiums paid. If you die, the insurance company must pay out. If you don't, they keep your premiums. What you have bought is the sure knowledge that in the case of your death, the company will pay the face value of your policy to your family.

Cash-value insurance. This type accommodates people who would like to be able to provide for their beneficiaries throughout their lifetime without periodically renewing the policy at a higher rate. The premium remains fixed. What happens is that in the early years of the policy the premiums are paying for insurance. As the fund you have paid into accumulates, the savings and interest becomes the larger part of the face value of the policy and the insurance, or the protection in case of your death, the smaller part. In other words, in the case of your death, as you grow older much of what your beneficiaries will be receiving back will be your own savings. That is all well and good except that the rate of interest is, in most cases, lower than you would receive from an ordinary savings account. Furthermore, according to Consumer Reports it is almost impossible to find out from the insurance companies what the rates are or have been.

Term insurance versus cash value

Term insurance costs about one sixth that of cash-value insurance. For example, at age 35 a doctor could buy $100,000 of renewable term insurance for less than $300 yearly premium from an insurance company. Cash value or ordinary life would cost about $1,800 for the same coverage. Since insurance is what we are talking about and not investment or savings, that is, pure financial protection in case of your death, term insurance is clearly the best buy. Although the cost of term insurance increases with the age of the insured, this can usually be offset by the changing circumstances of the family. In the average family the wife may go to work once the children are in school. Later, the children leave the nest, finish school, and are out on their own. At this point life insurance is scarcely needed.

Buying a term policy

Before calling your insurance agent, check into the rates of policies that might be available to you as a member of a group. But compare rates, if you have any choices. A group that consists of a majority of older people will have higher rates than a younger group. There may be other variations as well. In New York, Massachusetts, and Connecticut you can buy life insurance from savings banks, thus avoiding the high cost of the commissioned salesperson.

Such insurance may be somewhat less flexible because of legal restrictions, but is will be cheaper.

The term insurance you buy should be renewable until you are 65 years old. Consumer Reports recommends that it be convertible to a cash-value policy up until you are 60. You will probably not want to take advantage of this feature but you might need insurance for some reason at that time of your life.

RETIREMENT AND OLD AGE

Before any consideration of such traditional investments as real estate and corporate stocks and bonds, or such exotic ventures as oil wells or gold mines, the prudent investor, mindful of retirement and old age, will calculate Social Security benefits and investigate such government tax-shelter plans as Individual Retirement Accounts (IRA) and Keogh plans. As with life insurance the first step is to try to anticipate how much money you will need to live on during your retirement years. Social Security will form the basis for a retirement income but will scarcely prove sufficient. IRA and Keogh plans may make up a substantial part of the difference, depending upon your age at the inception of the plans. If you are now doing some part-time work as an employee, you may be eligible for a pension. A further source of income over the age of 65 is working. One of the advantages of private practice is that the practitioner is not forced to retire. The earnings from working two or three days a week can form a substantial part of a retirement income. The Social Security Administration has calculated the percentage of income derived from various sources of the average American (Table 9–3).

TABLE 9–3
Sources of income for Americans over the age of 65

Earnings from work	30 percent
Savings and investment	25
Social Security	26
Other public pensions	6
Private pensions	5
Veterans' benefits	3
Public assistance	3
Other sources	2
Total	100 percent

Working

Many private practitioners would not consider retiring at age 60 or 65. They are not forced to do so by employers and are still finding excitement and enthusiasm for work. However, they may begin to slow down, take a day or two off a week, and a month or so off in the winter. Dr. X, an optometrist, sold his store. He works two or three days a week doing eye examinations and prescriptions for a colleague who welcomes any time that Dr. X will work, and pays him generously. Working not only contributes to a retirement income, but contributes to the health and well-being of health practitioners, keeping them in touch with younger people and offering a sense of usefulness and purpose to their lives. A disadvantage of working is that until the practitioner reaches age 72, one dollar is deducted from Social Security benefits for every two dollars earned in excess of a yearly total of $6,000. After age 72 there is no penalty. There is no penalty either for unearned income, that is from dividends, rents, or interest.

Social Security

Social Security is a mammoth federal insurance plan for all Americans, with a few minor exceptions. Employees, employers, and self-employed people pay Social Security taxes (FICA). The benefits vary according to how much was paid into the fund and for how many years. The maximum retirement benefits as of the fall of 1982 are in the neighborhood of $700 a month. A spouse is entitled to one half of the benefits of the retired worker so that a practitioner and spouse may receive as much as $12,600 a year. A working spouse earning at the top of the scale may increase that amount to $16,800. A spouse has the choice of receiving benefits either at the rate of his or her own earnings or at half of the rate of the worker's earnings, but not both. The amounts are somewhat lower if you elect to start receiving payments at 62 and 1 percent higher for each year you remain working until the age of 72. Eligibility extends to divorced wives of retired workers if they were married for 10 years.

As you can see, Social Security rules and regulations are anything but cut and dried. Your benefits depend in the first place on proper reporting and payments by an employer or yourself. It is advised that you obtain a free postcard from your local Social Security office (listed in the phone book under United States government, Health, Education and Welfare) called "Request for Statement of Earnings" to ascertain that your records are in proper order. You will receive a statement of your earnings for the past three years. There is a time limit of 3 years, 3 months, and 15 days after the year in which you worked during which you may make corrections. You can request your local Social Security office to calculate your potential benefits from the Statement of Earnings. Since Social Security benefits are subject to change, it is advisable to check periodically with the local office to see if any changes apply to your own situation. You will not automatically receive checks from the government when you reach age 65, you must apply.

Individual Retirement Accounts (IRA) and Keogh plans

The federal government in recent years has devised an incentive to encourage people who are not covered by other pension or profit-sharing plans to put away money for their retirement. The Individual Retirement Account (IRA) and Keogh plans are essentially tax shelters, that is, both the money invested and the interest received are not immediately subject to federal income taxes. The idea is that you will not be taxed until you finally begin to distribute (withdraw) the money that has accumulated, when you are between the ages of 59.5 and 70. At that time you will presumably have a lower income so that you will be paying at a lower rate. The incentive, however, is an immediate one because you can save in taxes up to half of what you put into your retirement account because the amount is subtracted from your gross income when you calculate your federal income tax. For example, practitioners in the 50 percent bracket would have to earn $3,000 to invest $1,500 outside of their IRAs or Keoghs. IRAs and Keogh plans are really tailored to the needs of private practitioners who should make every effort to avail themselves of the opportunities presented.

The IRA. Any individual who is not an active member of a tax-qualified retirement plan or profit-sharing plan during the taxable year and is under 70.5 years of age is eligible for a high interest tax-deferred IRA. Your account may be with any or several of the following: commercial banks, savings and loan associations, insurance companies, money-market funds, mutual funds, and stock and bond brokerage houses. You can move an account from one institution to another without penalty.

You may contribute each year up to $2,000 to an IRA. If your spouse works, he or she may set up a separate IRA and also contribute up to $2,000. If your spouse does not work, you may contribute a total of $2,250 for both of you, in two separate accounts. As we said before, the entire contribution is deductible from your income tax and you do not pay any tax on the earnings. You cannot withdraw any money from the account until you are 59.5 years old, become disabled, or die, without paying taxes on the amount withdrawn and a penalty of 10 percent of the money distributed (withdrawn). You must begin distribution of the money before you are 70.5 or be subject to a penalty. For more information see IRS Publication 590, Tax Information on Individual Retirement Arrangements.

The advantage of an IRA over insurance or private retirement plans is that the administrative costs are little or nothing. Also, if you put the money into Certificates of Deposit at a bank or into a money market fund, you do not have to spend any time managing the money.

Keogh plans. For the older practitioner with money to invest, who is a sole proprietor or a partner, the principal advantage of a Keogh plan or a corporate retirement plan over an IRA is that more tax-sheltered money can be put away each year. You can put up to 15 percent of your income, but not more than $15,000 into a Keogh plan; but if you have any employees who have been working for you for more than three years, you must also make contributions for each employee working more than 20 hours a week at the same percentage of their income as your contribution to your own income. The contribution you make to a Keogh for an employee is, of course, a deductible expense. You have control of the investment of the Keogh fund but your employees may take their share with them on termination of their employment.

The money in a Keogh may be invested with banks in Certificates of Deposit, with money market or mutual funds, insurance companies or, in practice, any way you see fit. It pays to shop around for the best rate of interest as a point or two can amount to a considerable sum of money over the years. For more details see IRS Publication 560, Tax Information on Self-employed Retirement Plans.

IRAs can be shifted into Keogh plans when a practitioner begins to have more money to spare. The lesson for self-employed people is to start putting money away in a tax-sheltered IRA immediately. It is enforced savings but the tax advantages make it such a good deal that it is almost throwing money away not to take advantage of the saving.

If a private practitioner incorporates, then there are even greater possibilities for pension plans, but employees must be included at the same proportional rates. Consult your accountant, lawyer, or possibly your banker to determine when it becomes worthwhile to incorporate to take advantage of the tax-sheltered pension plans available to corporations.

Other investments

The money contributed to IRAs and Keogh plans is usually used to buy government bonds, Certificates of Deposit, or other safe and reliable securities. Real estate, particularly your own home, has been a good investment over the last 10 years. Owning your own office may also be a good investment if the location is a good one. Interestingly enough, the money markets have paid off at the best rate over the past 10 years as compared to real estate, corporate stocks and bonds, gold, silver, and the other commodities.

Health professionals are advised to invest in their own practices (Farber, 1981), a business with which they are intimately acquainted, before putting their money into ventures with which they are less familiar. The financial pages of the *New York Times, The Wall Street Journal,* the business magazines, and many best-selling books offer all kinds of advice to the investor. Be wary, careful, and avoid impulse buying. Do not allow yourself to be seduced by the time-share vacation apartment, the wildcat oil well, or any other scheme, without a good deal of thought as well as advice from experts you trust. Health professionals are particularly subject to being preyed upon by the less than scrupulous salesperson. The best advice is the time honored one, "Don't bet more than you can afford to lose."

10

Stress management

STRESS

A man comes into your office. He needs a physical exam because he is switching employers. He continually looks at his watch. "Say, can't you hurry this up, Doc? There's nothing wrong with me." You ask him what he does for a living. He's a cab driver, smokes a pack of cigarettes a day, hasn't bothered with breakfast since his divorce, grabs a hot dog for lunch in the cab. You take his blood pressure. It is 195/110. "A classic Type A," you say to yourself, "He's a candidate for early myocardial infarction." Driving a cab is one of the more stressful occupations. He is recently divorced and is changing companies—two of the more stressful of life events. And the smoking and poor nutrition will only increase his chances. "Poor guy," you say to yourself.

But what about yourself? Physicians (particularly surgeons) have a disproportionately high incidence of myocardial infarction with stress as a contributing factor (House, 1974). Other health practitioners may be just as susceptible because of the nature of their work. Many studies suggest that the jobs of high risk people generally entail a high degree of responsibility for others, comparatively high work loads, and role conficts among other stressors (cf. Jenkins, 1971), surely an apt description of a health professional with a busy practice. The health practitioner is subject to stress in a number of areas—the pressure of the work day, handling business and administrative problems as well as the clinical work, the interpersonal relationships on the job, and juggling the competing demands of job, personal life, and professional advancement.

The term stress is frequently used in ordinary conversation to refer to all sorts of difficulties—something that everyone feels from time to time. Researchers have identified stress with a variety of feelings and reactions: anxiety, intense emotional and physiological arousal, and frustration. It is thought to be brought on by a wide range of circumstances, most prevalently, conflict. Although stress may involve any or all of these things, it is possible to set stress apart as a concept in its own right, composed of a threat, called the stressor, and a response which consists of a measurable alteration of the physiology and/or the behavior of an individual. The stressors acting on the cab driver were the stressors of his job, his divorce, and his poor personal health patterns. The alteration in his physiology could be said to be high blood pressure.

Working hard is not stressful, nor will doing your best within clearly defined limits promote heart disease. What seems to create stress is a sense of working against insurmountable or continually surmounting odds, constantly trying to gain control of a situation, coping in a situation in which one feels limited. Stress is also related to change—routines that no longer work. For example, the death of a spouse is considered to be the most stressful of all life events, not only an event over which the surviving spouse has no control, but one that causes major changes in many aspects of the survivor's life (see Table 10–1).

TABLE 10-1
Social readjustment rating scale*

Rank	Life event	Mean value
1	Death of spouse	100
2	Divorce	73
3	Marital separation	65
4	Jail term	63
5	Death of close family member	63
6	Personal injury or illness	53
7	Marriage	50
8	Fired at work	47
9	Marital reconciliation	45
10	Retirement	45
11	Change in health of family member	44
12	Pregnancy	40
13	Sex difficulties	39
14	Gain of new family member	39
15	Business readjustment	39
16	Change in financial state	38
17	Death of close friend	37
18	Change to different line of work	36
19	Change in number of arguments with spouse	35
20	Mortgage over $10,000	31
21	Foreclosure of mortgage or loan	30
22	Change in responsibilities at work	29
23	Son or daughter leaving home	29
24	Trouble with in-laws	29
25	Outstanding personal achievement	28
26	Wife begin or stop work	26
27	Begin or end school	26
28	Change in living conditions	25
29	Revision of personal habits	24
30	Trouble with boss	23
31	Change in work hours or conditions	20
32	Change in residence	20
33	Change in schools	20
34	Change in recreation	19
35	Change in church activities	19
36	Change in social activities	18
37	Mortgage or loan less than $10,000	17
38	Change in sleeping habits	16
39	Change in number of family get-togethers	15
40	Change in eating habits	15
41	Vacation	13
42	Christmas	12
43	Minor violations of the law	11

*Social Readjustment Rating Scale ranks life events in descending order; highest values require greatest adaptation and are most likely to trigger disease.

Source: J. Solomon, "The Price of Change." *The Sciences* 11, no. 9 (November 1971), p. 29.

Stressors on the job

For health professionals the clinical work itself may be the severest of on-the-job stressors. A pediatrician has commented that clinically, pediatrics is the least stressful of the specialties. "Children," she said, "tend to get well." But many practitioners deal day after day with people who cannot be made well—people who die. This is an uncontrollable event despite the best that modern medicine has to offer.

Add to that the distorted expectations of the patient role unconsciously held by most practitioners, that patients are supposed to get better. And they are supposed to get better because of the intervention of the practitioner. Unconsciously we may wish for them to be grateful to us if they have recovered, or, at least minimally, to show their gratitude by the prompt payment of their bills. What may actually happen is that they don't get better, or if they do, they don't acknowledge that it is due to the practitioner's skill and care. They may or may not pay their bills, or after telling you how wonderful you are, not show up for their next appointment. At each of these junctures, your blood pressure and your pulse go up and you breathe faster—the physical signs of stress.

The daily routine in the delivery of health care has built-in stressors. An emergency in the morning can destroy the day's schedule, resulting in a circle of patients in the waiting room—an unmanageable situation. The need to return calls, keep patient records up-to-date, or take that extra few minutes to try to reassure someone who is frightened—all may press the practitioner beyond his or her ability to cope.

And there are undefined expectations to a private practice. Do you try to see everyone who asks for care? Do you really expect to help them all? Do you think you should be making more money than you do? Does your day become so overwhelming that you can't see how you will be able to provide the high quality of care your professionalism demands? With their own high standards often left unmet, many practitioners are deprived of the sense of satisfaction that comes with the successful completion of a difficult task. Instead, despite the miracles they may have wrought during the day, there is a feeling of frustration or even despair at what has *not* been done.

In addition to their clinical worries, private practitioners are businesspeople. They must be time managers—scheduling patients in a reasonable way so that the office can be run at a pace comfortable to the practitioner, staff, and patients. They must be financial managers supervising the financial cycle connected with a patient visit, i.e., getting paid—from explaining the bill and the charges, to collecting the fee.

Handling third-party payers is stressful since a large percentage of payments comes from these sources. A delay in payments has serious consequences for a practitioner's cash flow. The stress results from both the lack of direct control over the third-party payer and the loss of control resulting from a shortage of ready cash.

Private practitioners must be experts in public relations. How do you sell yourself to a new patient. How do you keep referrals from slipping through your fingers when they can always go down the street to Dr. X? How patients feel about you is important when you are in private practice.

Building your practice may be a source of stress. How can you control your professional image in the direction you have planned when you are dependent on those who happen to walk in your office door? Suppose you are a psychologist, particularly successful in dealing with anorexic and depressed adolescents, but are instead doing marriage counseling and treating alcoholics. You need the adults with emotional problems for your bread and butter but are having a difficult time getting adolescent referrals and are beginning to feel you are wasting your time. Your frustration becomes a stressor.

And, too, you may be a clinical and clerical supervisor having problems supervising the people who work in your office as well as several clinical assistants. You are frantic because your secretary in zealously keeping up on the typing and filing of patient records, neglected to send out an insurance form, setting back payments about three months. Supervision equals control. And when supervision gets out of control it is impossible to keep calm.

A final source of stress for ambitious young practitioners is the built-in conflict between practice and family, although this is not unique to the health professions. It is also a difficulty for businesspeople and other young professionals eager to make their mark. It may be particularly stressful for women working full time in the health professions to find the time and energy to bear children and care for them in their early years. Women as well as men suffer stress when caught between family and career.

Tell-tale signs of stress

"Well," you say, "some of the above situations certainly apply to my practice. But I'm pretty easygoing. I just attend to my patients and don't let all those petty details bother me too much." But perhaps your body is telling you things that you won't otherwise admit. The following are some typical signs of stress:

1. Are you sleepy on the job, perhaps in dealing with a particular patient or patients with a particular diagnosis?
2. Do you find your mind wandering or do you daydream in the above situations?
3. Are you always a little late, especially with certain patients? This could be a problem of time management but it also shows a reluctance to deal with specific situations.
4. Are you experiencing a change in your sleep patterns? Are you having trouble falling asleep or waking earlier than you would wish?
5. Have you increased your dependence on chemical aids either to relax or become stimulated? For example, are you drinking more coffee or using any other substance that alters the central nervous system such as alcohol, amphetamines, or cocaine? What about tranquilizers?

6. Are you irritable with your staff or members of your family?
7. Have you noticed a loss of creativity or interest in your practice?
8. Are you constantly preoccupied with work, talk about it socially, at home, or with anyone who will listen?

Any one of the above symptoms should draw your suspicions. Any combination of two would indicate that something was amiss.

HOW TO REDUCE STRESS

It has been said that the truly healthy or wise person can be defined as one who can live comfortably with an unresolved situation. Most of us are not that healthy. In the face of an unresolved conflict, for most of us, there are two possibilities: (1) resolve the conflict or (2) try to improve the ability to live with it. We can learn to live with stress by making stress-provoking situations more manageable.

The systems approach

Business systems help to reduce stress by turning potential crises into routines. For example, with the one-write system described in Chapters 7 and 8, the bookkeeping detail of the office is always under control. There are no loose ends. Everything is accounted for. You know to the penny what your bank balance shows. You know exactly how much is owed you, by whom, and what steps have been taken to collect unpaid accounts. You know that today third-party payers will be billed and tomorrow the bills for the month will be paid.

Management systems may seem burdensome at first, particularly if you are keeping the books yourself. And, perhaps, as you struggle through the figures at the end of a busy day, you will realize that for you to keep your sanity you need to hire someone else to keep the books. Systems keep your office not only managed but manageable. They will leave you free to attend to the more creative clinical aspects of your practice.

Policy formation

A patient who owes you less than $15 has been avoiding your calls. Your staff can't reach him. What to do? A drug salesperson is sitting in your office. You hate to waste her time. Should you fit in five minutes to listen to her before your next patient? You need a new copier. Which brand and model would best suit your needs? The choices can become overwhelming. If you have to treat every decision as a new and different problem, you have another source of stress on your hands.

Work out policies for handling recurring situations. For example, once you have established a policy about collections, seemingly stressful situations become routine. Suppose that you decide that you will not pursue a person beyond six months, and/or three letters and two phone calls, who owes you less than $20. After the stipulated time and contacts, the account is laid to rest in a file labeled uncollectible. As for salespeople, you can operate like the big department stores and set aside a specific time to see them, or decide not to see any at all, or whatever policy suits your practice. When it comes to buying items that cost, say, $100 or more, you will want to get the best value for your money. Maybe you really enjoy comparing items yourself, or you trust your secretary to find the best buy. Whatever policies you adopt, you will simplify your day and avoid raising your blood pressure by establishing a set of guidelines for commonly occurring predicaments, sticking to them, and possibly, if your practice is large enough to warrant it, keeping them in written form as a manual of office procedures and policies.

Time management

At some point an overachieving, busy professional must face up to the fact that he or she is only one person with exactly 24 hours each day available for work and life. Trying to squeeze in a little extra is a self-defeating tactic. The strategy must be to recognize your limitations. How many patients can you reasonably handle, giving each the attention he or she is paying for? How much time is required for the supervision of your administrative staff? Even if you have only one person working part time, some time must be allotted to giving directions, receiving messages, and checking on office details. What about remembering calls that have to be made, business appointments, carrying out plans?

One way to organize your time is with a time-management system. One such system is called the "Daytimer System" which is available in desk- or pocket-sized versions. The pocket version doubles as a wallet with compartments that include a diary that shows the week at glance; a pen (an absolute necessity when you are away from your desk); an address and phone book; notes "to be done today" that you can slip into the spiral binder of the diary; a place for your credit cards; and a place to hold and organize receipts (mileage, restaurant, gas).

Get into the habit of using a diary system for time management. You will find that you consult it frequently during the day. You will avoid the stress of panicking because of a forgotten phone call or a business detail you neglected to follow up. Again, the purpose is control—in this case, over your time.

Outside help

Stop inventing the wheel. You are not the first or only professional in private practice. Since stress is such a common complaint, many people have devised ways to keep their professional lives under control. Professional organizations often have formats whereby you may seek out people who appear to be not only successful, but possessed of an inner control—people who have confidence, who don't fluster or panic easily, who seem to have time. Ask them about their daily routine. How many patients do they see a week? How long do they spend with each patient? What arrangements do they have for limiting their commitments. How do they handle emergencies? Do they share commitments with another professional? What decision making do they delegate to the administrative people in their office? Ask, too, specifically, about strategies they may have for keeping their sanity? Although not all of the answers will seem suitable to you some will strike a sympathetic note.

Some people jog to relax—not to compete in a marathon but just to be alone, listening to their own breath. Some doctors have a talent for music and play in a community orchestra or are members of a string quartet that meets on a regular basis. Winston Churchill and Dwight Eisenhower were Sunday painters.

One way to avoid or reduce stress is to ally yourself with others. Don't try to go it alone—you against them. Look for help and look to give help and thereby feel that there are others you can count on when you need them. Even one other person, someone in your field whom you trust, can function as a confidant, a person who will understand your concerns and to whom you can turn when in doubt. You will also learn from listening as you ponder someone else's problems. Some people have been lucky enough to have had a mentor, an older person to steer them through the career passages. In turn, you may give a leg up to a student or a younger professional as you gain in wisdom and have personal favors you can call in.

Some private practitioners have formed study groups that meet on a regular basis to discuss common problems, both of a business and a clinical nature. Membership in such a group need not be confined to people in the same specialty. In a small group of congenial people you may find that others are bothered by exactly the same things that are troubling you. You can discuss problems that are really not of any interest to anybody except those who are in a similar situation.

Professional help

If running your office seems to be the principal cause of your impatience and anger, pay a consultant to analyze your business procedures. Find a consultant whose specialty is private medical practice. Your local professional society may be able to recommend a consultant in your area or you may find one in the Yellow Pages. Be sure to ask for references.

A business consultant, trained and experienced in private practice, is familiar with the problems you are having and will be able to set up systems to keep your business in order and under control. A consultant will probably not end up telling you very much you were not aware of already, but the mere fact that you have to pay for the advice may insure that you will be assiduous about following the management systems suggested.

Other professional help

You will need other professional help, such as an attorney and an accountant, two people on whom you can really rely and in whose judgment you will have confidence. Both of these professionals are people who will represent you and guide you in crisis situations, as well as offer advice in the everyday management of your practice. Some professionals make a crisis out of the ordinary and some are able to take the fear and anxiety out of a crisis. Needless to say, you will find the latter a less stressful person to consult.

Two other characteristics you should look for are (1) how you feel about them and (2) their accessibility. You will want to feel comfortable with your attorney and your accountant. You are far better off with a less prestigious or even less experienced person whom you trust and can talk to and whom you feel is listening and interested in you and your problems, than you are with a "big shot" to whom you feel unimportant. You have to be able to explain yourself and to understand the professional's message. The second point about accessibility is obvious. You want to be able to reach your lawyer and accountant when you need them, if not instantly, within reasonable call back time.

Personal growth

Suppose you find that you just cannot rid yourself of tension. All your bookkeeping systems are under control and your daily schedule is a shining example of time management, but you are jumpy, irritable, and harrassed. The stress may lie within. Perhaps there is an incongruence between your expectations and goals, and life's realities. You may want to go to a psychotherapist to talk about yourself, your personal relationships, and your work. Or you might want to participate in a week-end growth group. Telling a group of sympathetic strangers about your life and listening to them talk about their worries may give you some confidence and dispel your feelings of uniqueness and aloneness.

TAKING CARE OF YOUR BODY

A number of relaxation techniques have come to us from the Eastern tradition (see the next section). You can slow down your heart beat and lower your blood pressure by meditation. It is a specific stress reliever. Yoga exercises have the same effect and also keep your muscles in good tone and your body flexible.

Be good to your body. Good nutrition and exercise reduce stress. Moderate exercise on a regular basis is better than too strenuous or no exercise at all. Eat a good breakfast. Drink alcohol in moderation (not more than two drinks a day). Don't smoke. Get seven or eight hours of sleep a night. Keep weight off. Avoid salt, fats, and sugar.

RELAXATION TECHNIQUES

Autogenics

Lie or sit quietly. Breathe slowly. As you exhale, say one of the following phrases to yourself. Repeat the phrase eight times, then go on to the next one:

My arms and legs are heavy.

My arms and legs are warm.

My heart beat is calm and regular.

It breathes me.

My abdomen is warm.

My forehead is cool.

Practice several times a day in 15 minute sessions.

Meditation

Sit quietly in a comfortable position. Close your eyes. Deeply relax all your muscles beginning at your feet and progessing up to your face. Keep the muscles relaxed. Breathe through your nose. Become aware of your breathing, listening to it.

As you breathe out, say the word "one" silently to yourself. Breathe easily and naturally. If a thought comes to mind, examine it briefly and discard it. Continue for 10 to 20 minutes. When you finish, sit quietly for several minutes. Don't interact or fight with distracting thoughts. Return your attention to repeating the word "one."

Color and sound

The simple do-re-mi scale is said to tune up nerve centers along the spine. Next time you are in the shower, sound one long note per breath. When you get to the top of the scale, go back down again.

Aum (om) is a sound said to resonate with the earth itself. Sit quietly and inhale deeply through your nose. As you exhale, relax your throat and sing at whatever pitch feels effortless. The *aum* will vibrate in your throat and down your spine. Try another deep breath. Repeat the *aum* until you feel energized and satisfied.

Color has a vibratory way of influencing the body in a similar fashion to sound. Sit and breathe quietly. Imagine yourself basking in the following sequence of colors, allowing a few moments with each: red, orange, yellow, green, blue, indigo, violet, and white. Say to yourself: "I breathe in

_____ from the good air. _____ fills and surrounds me, nourishing every cell."

You may notice that while some colors are dull, others are brilliant. This depends on your mood and energy, and what your body needs to feel balanced.

Psychosomatics

Psychosomatics enables you to make peace between your mind and body by getting in touch with exactly what you need to feel better. It usually starts with taking time for yourself and focusing on what bothers you. You fantasize a script or a change, see a turn for the better, and feel better. For example, imagining shining knights winning a battle with confused creatures can acually help your immune system destroy a tumor. In essence, your thoughts can help to heal your body (*New Roots,* May 1982).

References

Brook, R. H. & Williams, K. N. Malpractice and the quality of care. *Annals of Internal Medicine,* 1978, *88,* 836.

Curran, W. J. The Malpractice Commission Report. *New England Journal of Medicine,* 1973, *288,* 1222.

Curran, W. J. Malpractice claims: New data and trends. *New England Journal of Medicine,* 1979, *300,* 26.

DeWitt, C. Can patient records be both private and accessible? *Hospitals,* August 16, 1981, pp. 87–90.

Farber, L. (Ed.). *Personal money management for physicians.* Oradell, N.J.: Medical Economics Co., 1981.

Fifer, W. R. Risk management and medical malpractice. *Quality Review Bulletin,* April 1979, pp. 9–13.

Friedman, E. Shifting sands: State laws redefine records accessibility. *Hospitals,* August 16, 1981, pp. 81-83.

Gehrman, R. E. Dentists on the move: Making changes for the better. *Dentalpractice,* July/August, 1981.

Gregg, J. E. *The health insurance racket and how to beat it.* Chicago: Henry Regnery Co., 1974.

Holder, A. R. The standard of care. *Journal of the American Medical Association,* 1973, *225,* 671; 791; 1027.

Holder, A. R. Medicolegal rounds: The importance of medical records. *Journal of the American Medical Association,* 1974, *228*(1), 115.

House, J. S. Occupation stress and coronary disease: A review and theoretical integration. *Journal of Health and Social Behavior,* March 1974, pp. 12–27.

Jenkins, C. D. Psychological and social precursors of coronary disease: I. *New England Journal of Medicine,* 1971, *284*(6), 244–55.

Life insurance. *Consumer Reports,* February 1980, pp. 79–91.

Malasanos, L., Barkauskas, V., Moss, M., Stoltenberg-Allen, K. *Health assessment.* St. Louis: C. V. Mosby Co., 1981.

Mortgage life insurance. *Consumer Reports,* May 1981, pp. 277–90.

Raus, E. E., & Raus, M. M. *Manual of history taking, physical examination and record keeping.* Philadelphia: Lippincott, 1974.

Reinhold, R. E. As physician supply swells, more doctors choose rural America. *New York Times,* July 27, 1982, p. C-1.

Richards, J. S. Here is second MSMS report on Michigan medical malpractice claims. *Michigan Medicine,* 1978, *77,* 272.

Ridgewood Financial Institute. *Guide to Private Practice.* Ridgewood, N.J., 1980.

Rubin, B. Medical malpractice suits can be avoided. *Hospitals,* 1978, *52,* 87.

Somers, H. M. The malpractice controversy and the quality of patient care. *Millbank Memorial Fund Quarterly,* 1977, *55,* 193.

Schwartz, W. B., and Komisar, N. K. Doctors, damages, and deterrence: An economic view of medical malpractice. *New England Journal of Medicine,* 1978, *298,* 1282.

U.S. Department of Health, Education and Welfare. Report of the Secretary's Commission on Medical Malpractice (Publication no. 78-88). Washington, D.C.: U.S. Printing Office, January 1973.

Vaccarino, J. M. Malpractice: The problem in perspective. *Journal of the American Medical Association,* 1977, *238,* 861.

Weed, L. L. Quality control and the medical record. *Archives of Internal Medicine,* 1971, *127,* 101-5.

Wright, R. H. What to do until the malpractice lawyer comes: A survivor's manual. *American Psychologist,* 1981, *36,* 1535.

Ziegler, A. B. *Patient record controls.* Oradell, N.J.: Medical Economics Co., 1979.

Annotated bibliography

Ackerman, D. L. *Getting rich: A smart woman's guide to successful money management*. New York: A & W Publishers, 1981.
An excellent guide to insurance, retirement, and investment for breadwinners of either sex.

American Medical Association. *American medical directory: Geographic register of physicians*, 27th ed. Chicago: American Medical Association, 1979; also *Update to the 27th edition*. Chicago: American Medical Association, 1981.
Physicians are listed according to the location where they practice. Information on each physician includes address, age, medical school, primary and secondary specialties, type of practice (i.e., direct patient care, administration, research, and so on) and specialty board.

County and city data book. U.S. Chamber of Commerce, Washington, D.C.
A complete statistical description of community facilities throughout the U.S.

Del Bueno, D. J. *A financial guide for nurses: Investing in yourself and others*. Boston: Blackwell Scientific Publications, 1981.
A collection of essays offering advice to guide nurses in making financial decisions: finding the right job, going on the lecture circuit, investing in education, insurance, and taxes are among the topics discussed.

Directory of medical specialties, 20th ed. Chicago: Marquis Who's Who, 1981–1982.
Information includes name, certification, birth date and place, education, career history, teaching positions, office address, and telephone number. Physicians listed are board certified. Listing is by geographic areas within each specialty.

Farber, L. *Personal money management for physicians*. Oradell, N.J.: Medical Economics Co., 1981.
A collection of articles that first appeared in *Medical Economics*. They are short, useful, well-written, making sense out of investment and tax issues.

Gorlick, S. H. (ed.) *The whys and wherefores of corporate practice*. Oradell, N.J.: Medical Economics Co., 1978.
Advice on incorporating a medical practice with a multitude of examples illustrating the fine points. Includes a survey of physicians who were asked questions concerning their experience with incorporation.

Gross, R. and Cullen, J. *Help: The basics of borrowing money*. New York: Times Books, 1980.
Helpful information and advice on when and how to go about borrowing money.

Innovative Cassette Programs. B.M.A. Audio Cassettes. 200 Park Avenue South, New York, New York 10003.

The publisher provides a wide spectrum of audio oriented programs to assist the practitioner. Included are such timely topics as helping cancer patients cope, self-directed assertiveness training, clinical hypnosis, and controlling depression. The materials are designed for practitioner and/or patient use, are well-thought out, and easy to administer and absorb. These programs have broad application for practice expansion.

Internal Revenue Service. Revised yearly. *Tax guide for small business: Income, excise, and employment taxes for individuals, partnerships, and corporations.* Publication 334. Available at local IRS offices. Free.

A most useful book, not only for preparing a tax return but for understanding the definitions and categories of activities of small businesses that are of interest to the IRS. A basic course in small business procedures from the point of view of the IRS. Read it whether or not you have an accountant prepare your income tax returns.

Mattera, M. C. *How to hire, train, and manage your employees.* Oradell, N.J.: Medical Economics Co., 1982.

Excellent guide to personnel management with an emphasis on worker satisfaction, tact, and good humor. Hard facts on salary levels, personnel manuals, and a good chapter on how to fire an employee.

Medical economics. A periodical devoted to the business aspects of private practice including personal finance, tax issues, as well as topics relevant for health practitioners, slanted toward the successful physician.

Medical and health information directory, 2d ed. Detroit: Gale Research Co., 1980.

A guide to state and national associations and agencies, grant sources, research centers, publications, private management consultants for health professionals and health agencies, and other information useful to health professionals.

Pressman, R. M. *Private practice: A handbook for the independent mental health practitioner.* New York: Gardner Press, 1979.

This guide contains much information for psychologists, counselors, and other psychotherapists in private practice. The author relies on his personal experience and insights, as well as the literature on the subject.

Psychotherapy Finances. Ridgewood Financial Institute, Inc. Box 509, Ridgewood, New Jersey 07451.

A must for any mental health practitioner. This monthly newsletter covers the whole spectrum of private practice issues giving timely advice on topics such as tax shelters, malpractice, and business expansion.

Quinn, J. B. *Everyone's money book.* New York: Delacorte Press, 1978.

The primary concern of this big book is personal finance—how to handle your money intelligently. The information re financial protection, i.e. health and life insurance, investment and social security regulations, is generous, accurate, and easy to understand.

Rabinowitz, P. M. *Talking medicine: America's doctors tell their own story.* New York: W. W. Norton, 1981.

A third year medical student, bewildered by his own career choices, talks to 25 doctors. They talk about their careers, their attitudes toward their practices, and many of the practical decisions they made re the financial and business aspects of private practice.

Rowland, H. S. (ed.) *The nurses almanac*. Germantown, Md.: Aspen Systems, 1978.
An "Information Please" almanac for nurses, bristling with statistics and fascinating information, much of it helpful in making career choices and financial decisions.

Schwartz, M. *Designing and building your own professional office*. Oradell, N.J.: Medical Economics Co., 1981.
For anyone thinking of building a professional office, constructing an office in an existing building, or remodeling an old building. Information includes plumbing, landscaping, etc. including the preliminary planning and cost estimates. Written by a dentist with first-hand experience.

The Small Business Reporter. *Avoiding management pitfalls*. San Francisco: Bank of America, 1977.

Small Business Administration.
The SBA has offices in most major cities and are a source of information about the business aspects of a private practice. Many of their publications are free or are available for a small sum.

Small Business Administration. *Business plan for small service firms*. Small Marketers Aid No. 153, 1979. Available at local SBA offices.
Emphasizes the necessity for an overall plan before you start up a service such as a health practice. Shows how to put together the pieces of a workable plan and what are some of the pitfalls.

Unthank, L. L. and Behrendt, H. M. *What you should know about individual retirement accounts*. Homewood, Ill.: Dow Jones-Irwin, 1978.
The format is question and answer and there is more detail than you might desire, but it is all there and the index will help you to find your own questions.

Vorzimer, L. H. *Using census data to select a store front*. Small Marketers Aid No. 154, 1974. Small Business Administration.
Available free from the field offices and Washington headquarters of SBA.
A pamphlet of instruction in interpreting census data.

Webster's medical office handbook. Springfield, Mass.: G. & C. Merriman Co., 1979.
The one reference that should be included in every private practitioners' library. This handbook is a quick and ready reference with answers to the myriad of questions that come up in day-to-day medical office management.

APPENDIX I

Codes of ethics for medicine, social work, psychology, psychiatry, and dentistry

A. American Medical Association Principles of Medical Ethics*

PREAMBLE

The medical profession has long subscribed to a body of ethical statements developed primarily for the benefit of the patient. As a member of this profession, a physician must recognize responsibility not only to patients, but also to society, to other health professionals, and to self. The following principles adopted by the American Medical Association are not laws, but standards of conduct which define the essentials of honorable behavior for the physician.

I. A physician shall be dedicated to providing competent medical service with compassion and respect for human dignity.

II. A physician shall deal honestly with patients and colleagues, and strive to expose those physicians deficient in character or competence, or who engage in fraud or deception.

III. A physician shall respect the law and also recognize a responsibility to seek changes in those requirements which are contrary to the best interests of the patient.

IV. A physician shall respect the rights of patients, of colleagues, and of other health professionals, and shall safeguard patient confidences within the constraints of the law.

V. A physician shall continue to study, apply, and advance scientific knowledge, make relevant information available to patients, colleagues, and the public, obtain consultation, and use the talents of other health professionals when indicated.

VI. A physician shall, in the provision of appropriate patient care, except in emergencies, be free to choose whom to serve, with whom to associate, and the environment in which to provide medical services.

VII. A physician shall recognize a responsibility to participate in activities contributing to an improved community.

Principles of Medical Ethics of the AMA (Chicago: American Medical Association, 1980). Reprinted with permission of the American Medical Association.

B.   Code of Ethics of the National Association of Social Workers*

PREAMBLE

This code is intended to serve as a guide to the everyday conduct of members of the social work profession and as a basis for the adjudication of issues in ethics when the conduct of social workers is alleged to deviate from the standards expressed or implied in this code. It represents standards of ethical behavior for social workers in professional relationships with those served, with colleagues, with employers, with other individuals and professions, and with the community and society as a whole. It also embodies standards of ethical behavior governing individual conduct to the extent that such conduct is associated with an individual's status and identity as a social worker.

This code is based on the fundamental values of the social work profession that include the worth, dignity, and uniqueness of all persons as well as their rights and opportunities. It is also based on the nature of social work, which fosters conditions that promote these values.

In subscribing to and abiding by this code, the social worker is expected to view ethical responsibility in as inclusive a context as each situation demands and within which ethical judgment is required. The social worker is expected to take into consideration all the principles in this code that have a bearing upon any situation in which ethical judgment is to be exercised and professional intervention or conduct is planned. The course of action that the social worker chooses is expected to be consistent with the spirit as well as the letter of this code.

In itself, this code does not represent a set of rules that will prescribe all the behaviors of social workers in all the complexities of professional life. Rather, it offers general principles to guide conduct, and the judicious appraisal of conduct, in situations that have ethical implications. It provides the basis for making judgments about ethical actions before and after they occur. Frequently, the particular situation determines the ethical principles that apply and the manner of their application. In such cases, not only the particular ethical principles are taken into immediate consideration, but also the entire code and its spirit. Specific applications of ethical principles must be judged within the context in which they are being considered. Ethical behavior in a given situation

---

*Code of Ethics of the National Association of Social Workers, (Washington, D.C.: NASW, July 1, 1980). Reprinted with permission from the National Association of Social Workers, Inc.

must satisfy not only the judgment of the individual social worker, but also the judgment of an unbiased jury of professional peers.

This code should not be used as an instrument to deprive any social worker of the opportunity or freedom to practice with complete professional integrity; nor should any disciplinary action be taken on the basis of this code without maximum provision for safeguarding the rights of the social worker affected.

The ethical behavior of social workers results not from edict, but from a personal commitment of the individual. This code is offered to affirm the will and zeal of all social workers to be ethical and to act ethically in all that they do as social workers.

The following codified ethical principles should guide social workers in the various roles and relationships and at the various levels of responsibility in which they function professionally. These principles also serve as a basis for the adjudication by the National Association of Social Workers of issues in ethics.

In subscribing to this code, social workers are required to cooperate in its implementation and abide by any disciplinary rulings based on it. They should also take adequate measures to discourage, prevent, expose, and correct the unethical conduct of colleagues. Finally, social workers should be equally ready to defend and assist colleagues unjustly charged with unethical conduct.

SUMMARY OF MAJOR PRINCIPLES

  I. The social worker's conduct and comportment as a social worker

    A. *Propriety.* The social worker should maintain high standards of personal conduct in the capacity or identity as social worker.

    B. *Competence and professional development.* The social worker should strive to become and remain proficient in professional practice and the performance of professional functions.

    C. *Service.* The social worker should regard as primary the service obligation of the social work profession.

    D. *Integrity.* The social worker should act in accordance with the highest standards of professional integrity.

    E. *Scholarship and research.* The social worker engaged in study and research should be guided by the conventions of scholarly inquiry.

  II. The social worker's ethical responsibility to clients

    F. *Primacy of clients' interests.* The social worker's primary responsibility is to clients.

    G. *Rights and prerogatives of clients.* The social worker should make every effort to foster maximum self-determination on the part of clients.

    H. *Confidentiality and privacy.* The social worker should respect trhe privacy of clients and hold in confidence all information obtained in the course of professional service.

    I. *Fees.* When setting fees, the social worker should ensure that they are fair, reasonable, considerate, and commensurate with the service performed and with due regard for the clients' ability to pay.

  III. The social worker's ethical responsibility to colleagues

    J. *Respect, fairness, and courtesy.* The social worker should treat colleagues with respect, courtesy, fairness, and good faith.

K. *Dealing with colleagues' clients.* The social worker has the responsibility to relate to the clients of colleagues with full professional consideration.

IV. The social worker's ethical responsibility to employers and employing organizations

L. *Commitments to employing organizations.* The social worker should adhere to commitments made to the employing organizations.

V. The social worker's ethical responsibility to the social work profession

M. *Maintaining the integrity of the profession.* The social worker should uphold and advance the values, ethics, knowledge, and mission of the profession.

N. *Community service.* The social worker should assist the profession in making social services available to the general public.

O. *Development of knowledge.* The social worker should take responsibility for identifying, developing, and fully utilizing knowledge for professional practice.

VI. The social worker's ethical responsibility to society

P. *Promoting the general welfare.* The social worker should promote the general welfare of society.

THE NASW CODE OF ETHICS

I. The social worker's conduct and comportment as a social worker

A. *Propriety—The social worker should maintain high standards of personal conduct in the capacity or identity as social worker.*

    1. The private conduct of the social worker is a personal matter to the same degree as is any other person's, except when such conduct compromises the fulfillment of professional responsibilities.

    2. The social worker should not participate in, condone, or be associated with dishonesty, fraud, deceit, or misrepresentation.

    3. The social worker should distinguish clearly between statements and actions made as a private individual and as a representative of the social work profession or an organization or group.

B. *Competence and professional development—The social worker should strive to become and remain proficient in professional practice and the performance of professional functions.*

    1. The social worker should accept responsibility or employment only on the basis of existing competence or the intention to acquire the necessary competence.

    2. The social worker should not misrepresent professional qualifications, education, experience, or affiliations.

C. *Service—The social worker should regard as primary the service obligation of the social work profession.*

    1. The social worker should retain ultimate responsibility for the quality and extent of the service that individual assumes, assigns, or performs.

    2. The social worker should act to prevent practices that are inhumane or discriminatory against any person or group of persons.

D. *Integrity—The social worker should act in accordance with the highest standards of professional integrity and impartiality.*

1. The social worker should be alert to and resist the influences and pressures that interfere with the exercise of professional discretion and impartial judgment required for the performance of professional functions.
2. The social worker should not exploit professional relationships for personal gain.

E. *Scholarship and research—The social worker engaged in study and research should be guided by the conventions of scholarly inquiry.*
1. The social worker engaged in research should consider carefully its possible consequences for human beings.
2. The social worker engaged in research should ascertain that the consent of participants in the research is voluntary and informed, without any implied deprivation or penalty for refusal to participate, and with due regard for participants' privacy and dignity.
3. The social worker engaged in research should protect participants from unwarranted physical or mental discomfort, distress, harm, danger, or deprivation.
4. The social worker who engages in the evaluation of services or cases should discuss them only for the professional purposes and only with persons directly and professionally concerned with them.
5. Information obtained about participants in research should be treated as confidential.
6. The social worker should take credit only for work actually done in connection with scholarly and research endeavors and credit contributions made by others.

II. The social worker's ethical responsibility to clients
F. *Primacy of clients' interests—The social worker's primary responsibility is to clients.*
1. The social worker should serve clients with devotion, loyalty, determination, and the maximum application of professional skill and competence.
2. The social worker should not exploit relationships with clients for personal advantage, or solicit the clients of one's agency for private practice.
3. The social worker should not practice, condone, facilitate or collaborate with any form of discrimination on the basis of race, color, sex, sexual orientation, age, religion, national origin, marital status, political belief, mental or physical handicap, or any other preference or personal characteristic, condition or status.
4. The social worker should avoid relationships or commitments that conflict with the interests of clients.
5. The social worker should under no circumstances engage in sexual activities with clients.
6. The social worker should provide clients with accurate and complete information regarding the extent and nature of the services available to them.
7. The social worker should apprise clients of their risks, rights, opportunities, and obligations associated with social service to them.

8. The social worker should seek advice and counsel of colleagues and supervisors whenever such consultation is in the best interest of clients.

9. The social worker should terminate service to clients, and professional relationships with them, when such service and relationships are no longer required or no longer serve the clients' needs or interests.

10. The social worker should withdraw services precipitously only under unusual circumstances, giving careful consideration to all factors in the situation and taking care to minimize possible adverse effects.

11. The social worker who anticipates the termination or interruption of service to clients should notify clients promptly and seek the transfer, referral, or continuation of service in relation to the clients' needs and preferences.

G. *Rights and prerogatives of clients—The social worker should make every effort to foster maximum self-determination on the part of clients.*

1. When the social worker must act on behalf of a client who has been adjudged legally incompetent, the social worker should safeguard the interests and rights of that client.

2. When another individual has been legally authorized to act in behalf of a client, the social worker should deal with that person always with the client's best interest in mind.

3. The social worker should not engage in any action that violates or diminishes the civil or legal rights of clients.

H. *Confidentiality and privacy—The social worker should respect the privacy of clients and hold in confidence all information obtained in the course of professional service.*

1. The social worker should share with others confidences revealed by clients, without their consent, only for compelling professional reasons.

2. The social worker should inform clients fully about the limits of confidentiality in a given situation, the purposes for which information is obtained, and how it may be used.

3. The social worker should afford clients reasonable access to any official social work records concerning them.

4. When providing clients with access to records, the social worker should take due care to protect the confidences of others contained in those records.

5. The social worker should obtain informed consent of clients before taping, recording, or permitting third party observation of their activities.

I. *Fees—When setting fees, the social worker should ensure that they are fair, reasonable, considerate, and commensurate with the service performed and with due regard for the clients' ability to pay.*

1. The social worker should not divide a fee or accept or give anything of value for receiving or making a referral.

III. The social worker's ethical responsibility to colleagues

J. *Respect, fairness, and courtesy—The social worker should treat colleagues with respect, courtesy, fairness, and good faith.*

1. The social worker should cooperate with colleagues to promote professional interests and concerns.

2. The social worker should respect confidences shared by colleagues in the course of their professional relationships and transactions.
3. The social worker should create and maintain conditions of practice that facilitate ethical and competent professional performance by colleagues.
4. The social worker should treat with respect, and represent accurately and fairly, the qualifications, views, and findings of colleagues and use appropriate channels to express judgments on these matters.
5. The social worker who replaces or is replaced by a colleague in professional practice should act with consideration for the interest, character, and reputation of that colleague.
6. The social worker should not exploit a dispute between a colleague and employers to obtain a position or otherwise advance the social worker's interest.
7. The social worker should seek arbitration or mediation when conflicts with colleagues require resolution for compelling professional reasons.
8. The social worker should extend to colleagues of other professions the same respect and cooperation that is extended to social work colleagues.
9. The social worker who serves as an employer, supervisor, or mentor to colleagues should make orderly and explicit arrangements regarding the conditions of their continuing professional relationship.
10. The social worker who has the responsibility for employing and evaluating the performance of other staff members, should fulfill such responsibility in a fair, considerate, and equitable manner, on the basis of clearly enunciated criteria.
11. The social worker who has the responsibility for evaluating the performance of employees, supervisees, or students should share evaluations with them.

K. *Dealing with colleagues' clients—The social worker has the responsibility to relate to the clients of colleagues with full professional consideration.*
   1. The social worker should not solicit the clients of colleagues.
   2. The social worker should not assume professional responsibility for the clients of another agency or a colleague without appropriate communication with that agency or colleague.
   3. The social worker who serves the clients of colleagues, during a temporary absence or emergency, should serve those clients with the same consideration as that afforded any client.

IV. The social worker's ethical responsibility to employers and employing organizations
L. *Commitments to employing organization—The social worker should adhere to commitments made to the employing organization.*
   1. The social worker should work to improve the employing agency's policies and procedures, and the efficiency and effectiveness of its services.
   2. The social worker should not accept employment or arrange student field placements in an organization which is currently under public sanction by NASW for violating personnel standards, or imposing limitations on or penalties for professional actions on behalf of clients.

3. The social worker should act to prevent and eliminate discrimination in the employing organization's work assignments and in its employment policies and practices.

4. The social worker should use with scrupulous regard, and only for the purpose for which they are intended, the resources of the employing organization.

V. The social worker's ethical responsibility to the social work profession

M. *Maintaining the integrity of the profession—The social worker should uphold and advance the values, ethics, knowledge, and mission of the profession.*

1. The social worker should protect and enhance the dignity and integrity of the profession and should be responsible and vigorous in discussion and criticism of the profession.

2. The social worker should take action through appropriate channels against unethical conduct by any other member of the profession.

3. The social worker should act to prevent the unauthorized and unqualified practice of social work.

4. The social worker should make no misrepresentation in advertising as to qualifications, competence, service, or results to be achieved.

N. *Community service—The social worker should assist the profession in making social services available to the general public.*

1. The social worker should contribute time and professional expertise to activities that promote respect for the utility, the integrity, and the competence of the social work profession.

2. The social worker should support the formulation, development, enactment, and implementation of social policies of concern to the profession.

O. *Development of knowledge—The social worker should take responsibility for identifying, developing, and fully utilizing knowledge for professional practice.*

1. The social worker should base practice upon recognized knowledge relevant to social work.

2. The social worker should critically examine, and keep current with emerging knowledge relevant to social work.

3. The social worker should contribute to the knowledge base of social work and share research knowledge and practice wisdom with colleagues.

VI. The social worker's ethical responsibility to society

P. *Promoting the general welfare—The social worker should promote the general welfare of society.*

1. The social worker should act to prevent and eliminate discrimination against any person or group on the basis of race, color, sex, sexual orientation, age, religion, national origin, marital status, political belief, mental or physical handicap, or any other preference or personal characteristic, condition, or status.

2. The social worker should act to ensure that all persons have access to the resources, services, and opportunities which they require.

3. The social worker should act to expand choice and opportunity for all persons, with special regard for disadvantaged or oppressed groups and persons.
4. The social worker should promote conditions that encourage respect for the diversity of cultures which constitute American society.
5. The social worker should provide appropriate professional services in public emergencies.
6. The social worker should advocate changes in policy and legislation to improve social conditions and to promote social justice.
7. The social worker should encourage informed participation by the public in shaping social policies and institutions.

C. Ethical Principles of Psychologists*

PREAMBLE

Psychologists respect the dignity and worth of the individual and strive for the preservation and protection of fundamental human rights. They are committed to increasing knowledge of human behavior and of people's understanding of themselves and others and to the utilization of such knowledge for the promotion of human welfare. While pursuing these objectives, they make every effort to protect the welfare of those who seek their services and of the research participants that may be the object of study. They use their skills only for purposes consistent with these values and do not knowingly permit their misuse by others. While demanding for themselves freedom of inquiry and communication, psychologists accept the responsibility this freedom requires: competence, objectivity in the application of skills, and concern for the best interests of clients, colleagues, students, research participants, and society. In the pursuit of these ideals, psychologists subscribe to principles in the following areas: 1. Responsibility, 2. Competence, 3. Moral and Legal Standards, 4. Public Statements, 5. Confidentiality, 6. Welfare of the Consumer, 7. Professional Relationships, 8. Assessment Techniques, 9. Research With Human Participants, and 10. Care and Use of Animals.

*Published by the American Psychological Association, 1200 Seventeenth Street, N.W., Washington, D.C. 20036. Copyright 1981 by the American Psychological Association. Reprinted by permission of the publisher and author.

This version of the Ethical Principles of Psychologists (formerly entitled Ethical Standards of Psychologists) was adopted by the American Psychological Association's Council of Representatives on January 24, 1981. The revised Ethical Principles contain both substantive and grammatical changes in each of the nine ethical principles constituting the Ethical Standards of Psychologists previously adopted by the Council of Representatives in 1979, plus a new tenth principle entitled Care and Use of Animals. Inquiries concerning the Ethical Principles of Psychologists should be addressed to the Administrative Officer for Ethics, American Psychological Association, 1200 Seventeenth Street, N.W., Washington, D.C. 20036.

These revised Ethical Principles apply to psychologists, to students of psychology, and to others who do work of a psychological nature under the supervision of a psychologist. They are also intended for the guidance of nonmembers of the Association who are engaged in psychological research or practice.

Any complaints of unethical conduct filed after January 24, 1981, shall be governed by this 1981 revision. However, conduct (a) complained about after January 24, 1981, but which occurred prior to that date and (b) not considered unethical under prior versions of the principles but considered unethical under the 1981 revision, shall not be deemed a violation of ethical principles. Any complaints pending as of January 24, 1981, shall be governed either by the 1979 or by the 1981 version of the Ethical Principles, at the sound discretion of the Committee on Scientific and Professional Ethics and Conduct.

Acceptance of membership in the American Psychological Association commits the member to adherence to these principles.

Psychologists cooperate with duly constituted committees of the American Psychological Association, in particular, the Committee on Scientific and Professional Ethics and Conduct, by responding to inquiries promptly and completely. Members also respond promptly and completely to inquiries from duly constituted state association ethics committees and professional standards review committees.

PRINCIPLE 1: RESPONSIBILITY

In providing services, psychologists maintain the highest standards of their profession. They accept responsibility for the consequences of their acts and make every effort to ensure that their services are used appropriately.

a. As scientists, psychologists accept responsibility for the selection of their research topics and the methods used in investigation, analysis, and reporting. They plan their research in ways to minimize the possibility that their findings will be misleading. They provide thorough discussion of the limitations of their data, especially where their work touches on social policy or might be construed to the detriment of persons in specific age, sex, ethnic, socioeconomic, or other social groups. In publishing reports of their work, they never suppress disconfirming data, and they acknowledge the existence of alternative hypotheses and explanations of their findings. Psychologists take credit only for work they have actually done.

b. Psychologists clarify in advance with all appropriate persons and agencies the expectations for sharing and utilizing research data. They avoid relationships that may limit their objectivity or create a conflict of interest. Interference with the milieu in which data are collected is kept to a minimum.

c. Psychologists have the responsibility to attempt to prevent distortion, misuse, or suppression of psychological findings by the institution or agency of which they are employees.

d. As members of governmental or other organizational bodies, psychologists remain accountable as individuals to the highest standards of their profession.

e. As teachers, psychologists recognize their primary obligation to help others acquire knowledge and skill. They maintain high standards of scholarship by presenting psychological information objectively, fully, and accurately.

f. As practitioners, psychologists know that they bear a heavy social responsibility because their recommendations and professional actions may alter the lives of others. They are alert to personal, social, organizational, financial, or political situations and pressures that might lead to misuse of their influence.

PRINCIPLE 2: COMPETENCE

The maintenance of high standards of competence is a responsibility shared by all psychologists in the interest of the public and the profession as a whole. Psychologists recognize the boundaries of their competence and the limitations of their techniques. They only provide services and only use techniques for which they are qualified by training and experience. In those areas in which recognized standards do not yet exist, psychologists take whatever precautions are necessary to protect the welfare of their clients.

They maintain knowledge of current scientific and professional information related to the services they render.

a. Psychologists accurately represent their competence, education, training, and experience. They claim as evidence of educational qualifications only those degrees obtained from institutions acceptable under the Bylaws and Rules of Council of the American Psychological Association.

b. As teachers, psychologists perform their duties on the basis of careful preparation so that their instruction is accurate, current, and scholarly.

c. Psychologists recognize the need for continuing education and are open to new procedures and changes in expectations and values over time.

d. Psychologists recognize differences among people, such as those that may be associated with age, sex, socioeconomic, and ethnic backgrounds. When necessary, they obtain training, experience, or counsel to assure competent service or research relating to such persons.

e. Psychologists responsible for decisions involving individuals or policies based on test results have an understanding of psychological or educational measurement, validation problems, and test research.

f. Psychologists recognize that personal problems and conflicts may interfere with professional effectiveness. Accordingly, they refrain from undertaking any activity in which their personal problems are likely to lead to inadequate performance or harm to a client, colleague, student, or research participant. If engaged in such activity when they become aware of their personal problems, they seek competent professional assistance to determine whether they should suspend, terminate, or limit the scope of their professional and/or scientific activities.

PRINCIPLE 3: MORAL AND LEGAL STANDARDS

Psychologists' moral and ethical standards of behavior are a personal matter to the same degree as they are for any other citizen, except as these may compromise the fulfillment of their professional responsibilities or reduce the public trust in psychology and psychologists. Regarding their own behavior, psychologists are sensitive to prevailing community standards and to the possible impact that conformity to or deviation from these standards may have upon the quality of their performance as psychologists. Psychologists are also aware of the possible impact of their public behavior upon the ability of colleagues to perform their professional duties.

a. As teachers, psychologists are aware of the fact that their personal values may affect the selection and presentation of instructional materials. When dealing with topics that may give offense, they recognize and respect the diverse attitudes that students may have toward such materials.

b. As employees or employers, psychologists do not engage in or condone practices that are inhumane or that result in illegal or unjustifiable actions. Such practices include, but are not limited to, those based on considerations of race, handicap, age, gender, sexual preference, religion, or national origin in hiring, promotion, or training.

c. In their professional roles, psychologists avoid any action that will violate or diminish the legal and civil rights of clients or of others who may be affected by their actions.

d. As practitioners and researchers, psychologists act in accord with Association standards and guidelines related to practice and to the conduct of research with human beings and animals. In the ordinary course of events, psychologists adhere to relevant governmental laws and institutional regulations. When federal, state, provincial, organizational, or institutional laws, regulations, or practices are in conflict with Association standards and guidelines, psychologists make known their commitment to Association standards and guidelines and, wherever possible, work toward a resolution of the conflict. Both practitioners and researchers are concerned with the development of such legal and quasi-legal regulations as best serve the public interest, and they work toward changing existing regulations that are not beneficial to the public interest.

PRINCIPLE 4: PUBLIC STATEMENTS

Public statements, announcements of services, advertising, and promotional activities of psychologists serve the purpose of helping the public make informed judgments and choices. Psychologists represent accurately and objectively their professional qualifications, affiliations, and functions, as well as those of the institutions or organizations with which they or the statements may be associated. In public statements providing psychological information or professional opinions or providing information about the availability of psychological products, publications, and services, psychologists base their statements on scientifically acceptable psychological findings and techniques with full recognition of the limits and uncertainties of such evidence.

a. When announcing or advertising professional services, psychologists may list the following information to describe the provider and services provided: name, highest relevant academic degree earned from a regionally accredited institution, date, type, and level of certification or licensure, diplomate status, APA membership status, address, telephone number, office hours, a brief listing of the type of psychological services offered, an appropriate presentation of fee information, foreign languages spoken, and policy with regard to third-party payments. Additional relevant or important consumer information may be included if not prohibited by other sections of these Ethical Principles.

b. In announcing or advertising the availability of psychological products, publications, or services, psychologists do not present their affiliation with any organization in a manner that falsely implies sponsorship or certification by that organization. In particular and for example, psychologists do not state APA membership or fellow status in a way to suggest that such status implies specialized professional competence or qualifications. Public statements include, but are not limited to, communication by means of periodical, book, list, directory, television, radio, or motion picture. They do not contain (*i*) a false, fraudulent, misleading, deceptive, or unfair statement; (*ii*) a misinterpretation of fact or a statement likely to mislead or deceive because in context it makes only a partial disclosure of relevant facts; (*iii*) a testimonial from a patient regarding the quality of a psychologist's services or products; (*iv*) a statement intended or likely to create false or unjustified expectations of favorable results; (*v*) a statement implying unusual, unique, or one-of-a-kind abilities; (*vi*) a statement intended or likely to appeal to a client's fears, anxieties, or emotions concerning the possible results of failure to obtain the offered services; (*vii*) a statement concerning the comparative desirability of offered services; (*viii*) a statement of direct solicitation of individual clients.

c. Psychologists do not compensate or give anything of value to a representative of the press, radio, television, or other communication medium in anticipation of, or in return for, professional publicity in a news item. A paid advertisement must be identified as such, unless it is apparent from the context that it is a paid advertisement. If communicated to the public by use of radio or television, an advertisement is prerecorded and approved for broadcast by the psychologist, and a recording of the actual transmission is retained by the psychologist.

d. Announcements or advertisements of "personal growth groups," clinics, and agencies give a clear statement of purpose and a clear description cf the experiences to be provided. The education, training, and experience of the staff members are appropriately specified.

e. Psychologists associated with the development or promotion of psychological devices, books, or other products offered for commerical sale make reasonable efforts to ensure that announcements and advertisements are presented in a professional, scientifically acceptable, and factually informative manner.

f. Psychologists do not participate for personal gain in commercial announcements or advertisements recommending to the public the purchase or use of proprietary or single-source products or services when that participation is based solely upon their identification as psychologists.

g. Psychologists present the science of psychology and offer their services, products, and publications fairly and accurately, avoiding misrepresentation through sensationalism, exaggeration, or superficiality. Psychologists are guided by the primary obligation to aid the public in developing informed judgments, opinions, and choices.

h. As teachers, psychologists ensure that statements in catalogs and course outlines are accurate and not misleading, particularly in terms of subject matter to be covered, bases for evaluating progress, and the nature of course experiences. Announcements, brochures, or advertisements describing workshops, seminars, or other educational programs accurately describe the audience for which the program is intended as well as eligibility requirements, educational objectives, and nature of the materials to be covered. These announcements also accurately represent the education, training, and experience of the psychologists presenting the programs and any fees involved.

i. Public announcements or advertisements soliciting research participants in which clinical services or other professional services are offered as an inducement make clear the nature of the services as well as the costs and other obligations to be accepted by participants in the research.

j. A psychologist accepts the obligation to correct others who represent the psychologist's professional qualifications, or associations with products or services, in a manner incompatible with these guidelines.

k. Individual diagnostic and therapeutic services are provided only in the context of a professional psychological relationship. When personal advice is given by means of public lectures or demonstrations, newspaper or magazine articles, radio or television programs, mail, or similar media, the psychologist utilizes the most current relevant data and exercises the highest level of professional judgment.

l. Products that are described or presented by means of public lectures or demonstrations, newspaper or magazine articles, radio or television programs, or similar media meet the same recognized standards as exist for products used in the context of a professional relationship.

PRINCIPLE 5: CONFIDENTIALITY

Psychologists have a primary obligation to respect the confidentiality of information obtained from persons in the course of their work as psychologists. They reveal such information to others only with the consent of the person or the person's legal representative, except in those unusual circumstances in which not to do so would result in clear danger to the person or to others. Where appropriate, psychologists inform their clients of the legal limits of confidentiality.

a. Information obtained in clinical or consulting relationships, or evaluative data concerning children, students, employees, and others, is discussed only for professional purposes and only with persons clearly concerned with the case. Written and oral reports present only data germane to the purposes of the evaluation, and every effort is made to avoid undue invasion of privacy.

b. Psychologists who present personal information obtained during the course of professional work in writings, lectures, or other public forums either obtain adequate prior consent to do so or adequately disguise all identifying information.

c. Psychologists make provisions for maintaining confidentiality in the storage and disposal of records.

d. When working with minors or other persons who are unable to give voluntary, informed consent, psychologists take special care to protect these persons' best interest.

PRINCIPLE 6: WELFARE OF THE CONSUMER

Psychologists respect the integrity and protect the welfare of the people and groups with whom they work. When conflicts of interest arise between clients and psychologists' employing institutions, psychologists clarify the nature and direction of their loyalties and responsibilities and keep all parties informed of their commitments. Psychologists fully inform consumers as to the purpose and nature of an evaluative, treatment, educational, or training procedure, and they freely acknowledge that clients, students, or participants in research have freedom of choice with regard to participation.

a. Psychologists are continually cognizant of their own needs and of their potentially influential position vis-à-vis persons such as clients, students, and subordinates. They avoid expliting the trust and dependency of such persons. Psychologists make every effort to avoid dual relationships that could impair their professional judgment or increase the risk of exploitation. Examples of such dual relationships include, but are not limited to, research with and treatment of employees, students, supervisees, close friends, or relatives. Sexual intimacies with clients are unethical.

b. When a psychologist agrees to provide services to a client at the request of a third party, the psychologist assumes the responsibility of clarifying the nature of the relationships to all parties concerned.

c. Where the demands of an organization require psychologists to violate these Ethical Principles, psychologists clarify the nature of the conflict between the demands and these principles. They inform all parties of psychologists' ethical responsibilities and take appropriate action.

d. Psychologists make advance financial arrangements that safeguard the best interests of, and are clearly understood by, their clients. They neither give nor receive any remuneration for referring clients for professional services. They contribute a portion of their services to work for which they receive little or no financial return.

e. Psychologists terminate a clinical or consulting relationship when it is reasonably clear that the consumer is not benefiting from it. They offer to help the consumer locate alternative sources of assistance.

PRINCIPLE 7: PROFESSIONAL RELATIONSHIPS

Psychologists act with due regard for the needs, special competencies, and obligations of their colleagues in psychology and other professions. They respect the prerogatives and obligations of the institutions or organizations with which these other colleagues are associated.

a. Psychologists understand the areas of competence of related professions. They make full use of all the professional, technical, and administrative resources that serve the best interests of consumers. The absence of formal relationships with other professional workers does not relieve psychologists of the responsibility of securing for their clients the best possible professional service, nor does it relieve them of the obligation to exercise foresight, diligence, and tact in obtaining the complementary or alternative assistance needed by clients.

b. Psychologists know and take into account the traditions and practices of other professional groups with whom they work and cooperate fully with such groups. If a person is receiving similar services from another professional, psychologists do not offer their own services directly to such a person. If a psychologist is contacted by a person who is already receiving similar services from another professional, the psychologist carefully considers that professional relationship and proceeds with caution and sensitivity to the therapeutic issues as well as the client's welfare. The psychologist discusses these issues with the client so as to minimize the risk of confusion and conflict.

c. Psychologists who employ or supervise other professionals or professionals in training accept the obligation to facilitate the further professional development of these individuals. They provide appropriate working conditions, timely evaluations, constructive consultation, and experience opportunities.

d. Psychologists do not exploit their professional relationships with clients, supervisees, students, employees, or research participants sexually or otherwise. Psychologists do not condone or engage in sexual harassment. Sexual harassment is defined as deliberate or repeated comments, gestures, or physical contacts of a sexual nature that are unwanted by the recipient.

e. In conducting research in institutions or organizations, psychologists secure appropriate authorization to conduct such research. They are aware of their obligations to future research workers and ensure that host institutions receive adequate information about the research and proper acknowledgment of their contributions.

f. Publication credit is assigned to those who have contributed to a publication in proportion to their professional contributions. Major contributions of a professional character made by several persons to a common project are recognized by joint authorship, with the individual who made the principal contribution listed first. Minor contributions of a professional character and extensive clerical or similar nonprofessional assistance may be acknowledged in footnotes or in an introductory statement. Acknowledgment through specific citations is made for unpublished as well as published material that has directly influenced the research or writing. Psychologists who compile and edit material of others for publication publish the material in the name of the originating group, if appropriate, with their own name appearing as chairperson or editor. All contributors are to be acknowledged and named.

g. When psychologists know of an ethical violation by another psychologist, and it seems appropriate, they informally attempt to resolve the issue by bringing the behavior to the attentiion of the psychologist. If the misconduct is of a minor nature and/or appears to be due to lack of sensitivity, knowledge, or experience, such an informal solution is usually appropriate. Such informal corrective efforts are made with sensitivity to any rights to confidentiality involved. If the violation does not seem amenable to an informal solution, or is of a more serious nature, psychologists bring it to the attention of the appropriate local, state, and/or national committee on professional ethics and conduct.

PRINCIPLE 8: ASSESSMENT TECHNIQUES

In the development, publication, and utilization of psychological assessment techniques, psychologists make every effort to promote the welfare and best interests of the client. They guard against the misuse of assessment results. They respect the client's right to know the results, the interpretations made, and the bases for their conclusions and recommendations. Psychologists make every effort to maintain the security of tests and other assessment techniques within limits of legal mandates. They strive to ensure the appropriate use of assessment techniques by others.

a. In using assessment techniques, psychologists respect the right of clients to have full explanations of the nature and purpose of the techniques in language the clients can understand, unless an explicit exception to this right has been agreed upon in advance. When the explanations are to be provided by others, psychologists establish procedures for ensuring the adequacy of these explanations.

b. Psychologists responsible for the development and standardization of psychological tests and other assessment techniques utilize established scientific procedures and observe the relevant APA standards.

c. In reporting assessment results, psychologists indicate any reservations that exist regarding validity or reliability because of the circumstances of the assessment or the inappropriateness of the norms for the person tested. Psychologists strive to ensure that the results of assessments and their interpretations are not misused by others.

d. Psychologists recognize that assessment results may become obsolete. They make every effort to avoid and prevent the misuse of obsolete measures.

e. Psychologists offering scoring and interpretation services are able to produce appropriate evidence for the validity of the programs and procedures used in arriving at interpretations. The public offering of an automated interpretation service is considered a professional-to-professional consultation. Psychologists make every effort to avoid misuse of assessment reports.

f. Psychologists do not encourage or promote the use of psychological assessment techniques by inappropriately trained or otherwise unqualified persons through teaching, sponsorship, or supervision.

PRINCIPLE 9: RESEARCH WITH HUMAN PARTICIPANTS

The decision to undertake research rests upon a considered judgment by the individual psychologist about how best to contribute to psychological science and human welfare. Having made the decision to conduct research, the psychologist considers alternative directions in which research energies and resources might be invested. On the basis of this consideration, the psychologist carries out the investigation with respect and concern for the dignity and welfare of the people who participate and with cognizance of federal and state regulations and professional standards governing the conduct of research with human participants.

a. In planning a study, the investgator has the responsibility to make a careful evaluation of its ethical acceptability. To the extent that the weighing of scientific and human values suggests a compromise of any principle, the investigator incurs a correspondingly serious obligation to seek ethical advice and to observe stringent safeguards to protect the rights of human participants.

b. Considering whether a participant in a planned study will be a "subject at risk" or a "subject at minimal risk," according to recognized standards, is of primary ethical concern to the investigator.

c. The investigator always retains the responsibility for ensuring ethical practice in research. The investigator is also responsible for the ethical treatment of research participants by collaborators, assistants, students, and employees, all of whom, however, incur similar obligations.

d. Except in minimal-risk research, the investigator establishes a clear and fair agreement with research participants, prior to their participation, that clarifies the obligations and responsibilities of each. The investigator has the obligation to honor all promises and commitments included in that agreement. The investigator informs the participants of all aspects of the research that might reasonably be expected to influence willingness to participate and explains all other aspects of the research about which the participants inquire. Failure to make full disclosure prior to obtaining informed consent requires additional safeguards to protect the welfare and dignity of the research particpants. Research with children or with participants who have impairments that would limit understanding and/or communication requires special safeguarding procedures.

e. Methodological requirements of a study may make the use of concealment or deception necessary. Before conducting such a study, the investigator has a special responsibility to (*i*) determine whether the use of such techniques is justified by the study's prospective scientific, educational, or applied value; (*ii*) determine whether alternative procedures are available that do not use concealment or deception; and (*iii*) ensure that the participants are provided with sufficient explanation as soon as possible.

f. The investigator respects the individual's freedom to decline to participate in or to withdraw from the research at any time. The obligation to protect this freedom requires careful thought and consideration when the investigator is in a position of authority or influence over the participant. Such positions of authority include, but are not limited to, situations in which research participation is required as part of employment or in which the particpant is a student, client, or employee of the investigator.

g. The investigator protects the participant from physical and mental discomfort, harm, and danger that may arise from research procedures. If risks of such consequences exist, the investigator informs the participant of that fact. Research procedures likely to cause serious or lasting harm to a participant are not used unless the failure to use these procedures might expose the participant to risk of greater harm, or unless the research has great potential benefit and fully informed and voluntary consent is obtained from each participant. The participant should be informed of procedures for contacting the investigator within a reasonable time period following participation should stress, potential harm, or related questions or concerns arise.

h. After the data are collected, the investigator provides the participant with information about the nature of the study and attempts to remove any misconceptions that may have arisen. Where scientific or humane values justify delaying or withholding this information, the investigator incurs a special responsibility to monitor the research and to ensure that there are no damaging consequences for the participant.

i. Where research procedures result in undesirable consequences for the individual participant, the investigator has the responsibility to detect and remove or correct these consequences, including long-term effects.

j. Information obtained about a research participant during the course of an investigation is confidential unless otherwise agreed upon in advance. When the possibility exists that others may obtain access to such information, this possibility, together with the plans for protecting confidentiality, is explained to the participant as part of the procedure for obtaining informed consent.

PRINCIPLE 10: CARE AND USE OF ANIMALS

An investigator of animal behavior strives to advance understanding of basic behavioral principles and/or to contribute to the improvement of human health and welfare. In seeking these ends, the investigator ensures the welfare of animals and treats them humanely. Laws and regulations notwithstanding, an animal's immediate protection depends upon the scientist's own conscience.

a. The acquisition, care, use, and disposal of all animals are in compliance with current federal, state or provincial, and local laws and regulations.

b. A psychologist trained in research methods and experienced in the care of laboratory animals closely supervises all procedures involving animals and is responsible for ensuring appropriate consideration of their comfort, health, and humane treatment.

c. Psychologists ensure that all individuals using animals under their supervision have received explicit instruction in experimental methods and in the care, maintenance, and handling of the species being used. Responsibilities and activities of individuals participating in a research project are consistent with their respective competencies.

d. Psychologists make every effort to minimize discomfort, illness, and pain of animals. A procedure subjecting animals to pain, stress, or privation is used only when an alternative procedure is unavailable and the goal is justified by its prospective scientific, educational, or applied value. Surgical procedures are performed under appropriate anesthesia; techniques to avoid infection and minimize pain are followed during and after surgery.

e. When it is appropriate that the animal's life be terminated, it is done rapidly and painlessly.

D. The Principles of Medical Ethics with Annotations Especially Applicable to Psychiatry*

FOREWORD

All physicians should practice in accordance with the medical code of ethics set forth in the Principles of Medical Ethics of the American Medical Association. An up-to-date expression and elaboration of these statements is found in the *Opinions and Reports of the Judicial Council* of the American Medical Association.[1] Psychiatrists are strongly advised to be familiar with these documents.[2]

However, these general guidelines have sometimes been difficult to interpret for psychiatry, so further annotations to the basic principles are offered in this document. While psychiatrists have the same goals as all physicians, there are special ethical problems in psychiatric practice that differ in coloring and degree from ethical problems in other branches of medical practice, even though the basic principles are the same. The annotations are not designed as absolutes and will be revised from time to time so as to be applicable to current practices and problems.

Following are the AMA Principles of Medical Ethics, printed in their entirety, and then each principle printed separately along with an annotation especially applicable to psychiatry.

PREAMBLE

The medical profession has long subscribed to a body of ethical statements developed primarily for the benefit of the patient. As a member of this profession, a physician must recognize responsibility not only to patients, but also to society, to other health profes-

---

*American Psychiatric Association, *The Principles of Medical Ethics* (Washington, D.C.: APA, 1981). Reprinted with permission of the American Psychiatric Association.

[1]*Opinions and Reports of the Judicial Council* (Chicago: American Medical Association, 1981).

[2]Chapter 8, Section 1 of the By-Laws of the American Psychiatric Association states, "All members of the American Psychiatric Association shall be bound by the ethical code of the medical profession, specifically defined in the *Principles of Medical Ethics* of the American Medical Association." In interpreting the APA Constitution and By-Laws, it is the opinion of the Board of Trustees that inactive status in no way removes a physician member from responsibility to abide by the *Principles of Medical Ethics*.

sionals, and to self. The following Principles, adopted by the American Medical Association, are not laws, but standards of conduct which define the essentials of honorable behavior for the physician.

Section 1

A physician shall be dedicated to providing competent medical service with compassion and respect for human dignity.

Section 2

A physician shall deal honestly with patients and colleagues, and strive to expose those physicians deficient in character or competence, or who engage in fraud or deception.

Section 3

A physician shall respect the law and also recognize a responsibility to seek changes in those requirements which are contrary to the best interests of the patient.

Section 4

A physician shall respect the rights of patients, of colleagues, and of other health professionals, and shall safeguard patient confidences within the constraints of the law.

Section 5

A physician shall continue to study, apply, and advance scientific knowledge, make relevant information available to patients, colleagues, and the public, obtain consultation, and use the talents of other health professionals when indicated.

Section 6

A physician shall, in the provision of appropriate patient care, except in emergencies, be free to choose whom to serve, with whom to associate, and the environment in which to provide medical services.

Section 7

A physician shall recognize a responsibility to participate in activities contributing to an improved community.

PRINCIPLES WITH ANNOTATIONS

Following are each of the AMA Principles of Medical Ethics printed separately along with annotations especially applicable to psychiatry.

PREAMBLE

The medical profession has long subscribed to a body of ethical statements developed primarily for the benefit of the patient. As a member of this profession, a physician must recognize responsibility not only to patients, but also to society, to other health professionals, and to self. The following Principles, adopted by the American Medical Association, are not laws, but standards of conduct which define the essentials of honorable behavior for the physician.

Section 1

A physician shall be dedicated to providing competent medical service with compassion and respect for human dignity.

1. The patient may place his/her trust in his/her psychiatrist knowing that the psychiatrist's ethics and professional responsibilities preclude him/her gratifying his/her own needs by exploiting the patient. This becomes particularly important because of the essentially private, highly personal, and sometimes intensely emotional nature of the relationship established with the psychiatrist.

2. A psychiatrist should not be a party to any type of policy that excludes, segregates, or demeans the dignity of any patient because of ethnic origin, race, sex, creed, age, socioeconomic status, or sexual orientation.

3. In accord with the requirements of law and accepted medical practice, it is ethical for a physician to submit his/her work to peer review and to the ultimate authority of the medical staff executive body and the hospital administration and its governing body. In case of dispute, the ethical psychiatrist has the following steps available:

a. Seek appeal from the medical staff decision to a joint conference committee, including members of the medical staff executive committee and the executive committee of the governing board. At this appeal, the ethical psychiatrist could request that outside opinions be considered.

b. Appeal to the governing body itself.

c. Appeal to state agencies regulating licensure of hospitals if, in the particular state, they concern themselves with matters of professional competency and quality of care.

d. Attempt to educate colleagues through development of research projects and data and presentations at professional meetings and in professional journals.

e. Seek redress in local courts, perhaps through an enjoining injunction against the governing body.

f. Public education as carried out by an ethical psychiatrist would not utilize appeals based solely upon emotion, but would be presented in a professional way and without any potential exploitation of patients through testimonials.

4. A psychiatrist should not be a participant in a legally authorized execution.

Section 2

A physician shall deal honestly with patients and colleagues, and strive to expose those physicians deficient in character or competence, or who engage in fraud or deception.

1. The requirement that the physician conduct himself with propriety in his/her profession and in all the actions of his/her life is especially important in the case of the psychiatrist because the patient tends to model his/her behavior after that of his/her therapist by identification. Further, the necessary intensity of the therapeutic relationship may tend to activate sexual and other needs and fantasies on the part of both patient and therapist, while weakening the objectivity necessary for control. Sexual activity with a patient is unethical.

2. The psychiatrist should diligently guard against exploiting information furnished by the patient and should not use the unique position of power afforded him/her by the psychotherapeutic situation to influence the patient in any way not directly relevant to the treatment goals.

3. A psychiatrist who regularly practices outside his/her area of professional competence should be considered unethical. Determination of professional competence should be made by peer review boards or other appropriate bodies.

4. Special consideration should be given to those psychiatrists who, because of mental illness, jeopardize the welfare of their patients and their own reputations and practices. It is ethical, even encouraged, for another psychiatrist to intercede in such situations.

5. Psychiatric services, like all medical services, are dispensed in the context of a contractual arrangement between the patient and the treating physician. The provisions of the contractual arrangement, which are binding on the physician as well as on the patient, should be explicitly established.

6. It is ethical for the psychiatrist to make a charge for a missed appointment when this falls within the terms of the specific contractual agreement with the patient. Charging for a missed appointment or for one not cancelled 24 hours in advance need not, in itself, be considered unethical if a patient is fully advised that the physician will make such a charge. The practice, however, should be resorted to infrequently and always with the utmost consideration of the patient and his/her circumstances.

7. An arrangement in which a psychiatrist provides supervision or administration to other physicians or nonmedical persons for a percentage of their fees or gross income is not acceptable; this would constitute fee-splitting. In a team of practitioners, or a multidisciplinary team, it is ethical for the psychiatrist to receive income for administration, research, education, or consultation. This should be based upon a mutually agreed upon and set fee or salary, open to renegotiation when a change in the time demand occurs. (See also Section 5, Annotations 2, 3, and 4.)

8. When a member has been found to have behaved unethically by the American Psychiatric Association or one of its constituent district branches, there should not be automatic reporting to the local authorities responsible for medical licensure, but the decision to report should be decided upon the merits of the case.

Section 3

A physician shall respect the law and also recognize a responsibility to seek changes in those requirements which are contrary to the best interests of the patient.

1. It would seem self-evident that a psychiatrist who is a lawbreaker might be ethically unsuited to practice his/her profession. When such illegal activities bear directly upon his/her practice, this would obviously be the case. However, in other instances,

illegal activities such as those concerning the right to protest social injustices might not bear on either the image of the psychiatrist or the ability of the specific psychiatrist to treat his/her patient ethically and well. While no committee or board could offer prior assurance that any illegal activity would not be considered unethical, it is conceivable that an individual could violate a law without being guilty of professionally unethical behavior. Physicians lose no right of citizenship on entry into the profession of medicine.

2. Where not specifically prohibited by local laws governing medical practice, the practice of acupuncture by a psychiatrist is not unethical per se. The psychiatrist should have professional competence in the use of acupuncture. Or, if he/she is supervising the use of acupuncture by nonmedical individuals, he/she should provide proper medical supervision. (See also Section 5, Annotations 3 and 4.)

Section 4

A physician shall respect the rights of patients, of colleagues, and of other health professionals, and shall safeguard patient confidences within the constraints of the law.

1. Psychiatric records, including even the identification of a person as a patient, must be protected with extreme care. Confidentiality is essential to psychiatric treatment. This is based in part on the special nature of psychiatric therapy as well as on the traditional ethical relationship between physician and patient. Growing concern regarding the civil rights of patients and the possible adverse effects of computerization, duplication equipment, and data banks makes the dissemination of confidential information an increasing hazard. Because of the sensitive and private nature of the information with which the psychiatrist deals, he/she must be circumspect in the information that he/she chooses to disclose to others about a patient. The welfare of the patient must be a continuing consideration.

2. A psychiatrist may release confidential information only with the authorization of the patient or under proper legal compulsion. The continuing duty of the psychiatrist to protect the patient includes fully apprising him/her of the connotations of waiving the privilege of privacy. This may become an issue when the patient is being investigated by a government agency, is applying for a position, or is involved in legal action. The same principles apply to the release of information concerning treatment to medical departments of government agencies, business organizations, labor unions, and insurance companies. Information gained in confidence about patients seen in student health services should not be released without the student's explicit permission.

3. Clinical and other materials used in teaching and writing must be adequately disguised in order to preserve the anonymity of the individuals involved.

4. The ethical responsibility of maintaining confidentiality holds equally for the consultations in which the patient may not have been present and in which the consultee was not a physician. In such instances, the physician consultant should alert the consultee to his/her duty of confidentiality.

5. Ethically the psychiatrist may disclose only that information which is relevant to a given situation. He/she should avoid offering speculation as fact. Sensitive information such as an individual's sexual orientation or fantasy material is usually unnecessary.

6. Psychiatrists are often asked to examine individuals for security purposes, to determine suitability for various jobs, and to determine legal competence. The psychiatrist

must fully describe the nature and purpose and lack of confidentiality of the examination to the examinee at the beginning of the examination.

7. Careful judgment must be exercised by the psychiatrist in order to include, when appropriate, the parents or guardian in the treatment of a minor. At the same time the psychiatrist must assure the minor proper confidentiality.

8. Psychiatrists at times may find it necessary, in order to protect the patient or the community from imminent danger, to reveal confidential information disclosed by the patient.

9. When the psychiatrist is ordered by the court to reveal the confidences entrusted to him/her by patients he/she may comply or he/she may ethically hold the right to dissent within the framework of the law. When the psychiatrist is in doubt, the right of the patient to confidentiality and, by extension, to unimpaired treatment, should be given priority. The psychiatrist should reserve the right to raise the question of adequate need for disclosure. In the event that the necessity for legal disclosure is demonstrated by the court, the psychiatrist may request the right to disclosure of only that information which is relevant to the legal question at hand.

10. With regard for the person's dignity and privacy and with truly informed consent, it is ethical to present a patient to a scientific gathering, if the confidentiality of the presentation is understood and accepted by the audience.

11. It is ethical to present a patient or former patient to a public gathering or to the news media only if that patient is fully informed of enduring loss of confidentiality, is competent, and consents in writing without coercion.

12. When involved in funded research, the ethical psychiatrist will advise human subjects of the funding source, retain his/her freedom to reveal data and results, and follow all appropriate and current guidelines relative to human subject protection.

13. Ethical considerations in medical practice preclude the psychiatric evaluation of any adult charged with criminal acts prior to access to, or availability of, legal counsel. The only exception is the rendering of care to the person for the sole purpose of medical treatment.

Section 5

A physician shall continue to study, apply, and advance scientific knowledge, make relevant information available to patients, colleagues, and the public, obtain consultation, and use the talents of other health professionals when indicated.

1. Psychiatrists are responsible for their own continuing education and should be mindful of the fact that theirs must be a lifetime of learning.

2. In the practice of his/her specialty, the psychiatrist consults, associates, collaborates, or integrates his/her work with that of many professionals, including psychologists, psychometricians, social workers, alcoholism counselors, marriage counselors, public health nurses, etc. Furthermore, the nature of modern psychiatric practice extends his/her contacts to such people as teachers, juvenile and adult probation officers, attorneys, welfare workers, agency volunteers, and neighborhood aides. In referring patients for treatment, counseling, or rehabilitation to any of these practitioners, the psychiatrist should ensure that the allied professional or paraprofessional with whom he/she is dealing is a recognized member of his/her own discipline and is competent to carry out the therapeutic task required. The psychiatrist should have the same attitude

toward members of the medical profession to whom he/she refers patients. Whenever he/she has reason to doubt the training, skill, or ethical qualifications of the allied professional, the psychiatrist should not refer cases to him/her.

3. When the psychiatrist assumes a collaborative or supervisory role with another mental health worker, he/she must expend sufficient time to assure that proper care is given. It is contrary to the interests of the patient and to patient care if he/she allows himself/herself to be used as a figurehead.

4. In relationships between psychiatrists and practicing licensed psychologists, the physician should not delegate to the psychologist or, in fact, to any nonmedical person any matter requiring the exercise of professional medical judgment.

5. The psychiatrist should agree to the request of a patient for consultation or to such a request from the family of an incompetent or minor patient. The psychiatrist may suggest possible consultants, but the patient or family should be given free choice of the consultant. If the psychiatrist disapproves of the professional qualifications of the consultant or if there is a difference of opinion that the primary therapist cannot resolve, he/she may, after suitable notice, withdraw from the case. If this disagreement occurs within an institution or agency framework, the differences should be resolved by the mediation or arbitration of higher professional authority within the institution or agency.

Section 6

A physician shall, in the provision of appropriate patient care, except in emergencies, be free to choose whom to serve, with whom to associate, and the environment in which to provide medical services.

1. Physicians generally agree that the doctor-patient relationship is such a vital factor in effective treatment of the patient that preservation of optimal conditions for development of a sound working relationship between a doctor and his/her patient should take precedence over all other considerations. Professional courtesy may lead to poor psychiatric care for physicians and their families because of embarrassment over the lack of a complete give-and-take contract.

Section 7

A physician shall recognize a responsibility to participate in activities contributing to an improved community.

1. Psychiatrists should foster the cooperation of those legitimately concerned with the medical, psychological, social, and legal aspects of mental health and illness. Psychiatrists are encouraged to serve society by advising and consulting with the executive, legislative, and judiciary branches of the government. A psychiatrist should clarify whether he/she speaks as an individual or as a representative of an organization. Furthermore, psychiatrists should avoid cloaking their public statements with the authority of the profession (e.g., "Psychiatrists know that . . .").

2. Psychiatrists may interpret and share with the public their expertise in the various psychosocial issues that may affect mental health and illness. Psychiatrists should always be mindful of their separate roles as dedicated citizens and as experts in psychological medicine.

3. On occasion psychiatrists are asked for an opinion about an individual who is in

the light of public attention, or who has disclosed information about himself/herself through public media. It is unethical for a psychiatrist to offer a professional opinion unless he/she has conducted an examination and has been granted proper authorization for such a statement.

4. The psychiatrist may permit his/her certification to be used for the involuntary treatment of any person only following his/her personal examination of that person. To do so, he/she must find that the person, because of mental illness, cannot form a judgment as to what is in his/her own best interests and that, without such treatment, substantial impairment is likely to occur to the person or others.

PROCEDURES FOR HANDLING COMPLAINTS OF UNETHICAL CONDUCT[3]

A complaint concerning the behavior of a member of this Association shall be in writing, signed by the complainant, and filed with the secretary. The secretary shall refer it to the appropriate District Branch for investigation and action. The secretary shall notify the accused member of the receipt of such a complaint and that it has been forwarded to the member's local District Branch and shall inform the accused member of his or her right to appeal any forthcoming action to the board. The District Branch may appeal to the Board for relief from responsibility for considering any complaint. The member against whom the complaint was brought shall have the right of appeal to the board for reconsideration of the decision of the District Branch.[4]

As noted above, a complaint must be written, must be signed by the complainant, and must be filed with the secretary of the Association.

Procedure A. Allegation received by District Branch

I. District Branch:
   A. Receives signed communication alleging or inferring unethical conduct.
   B. Determines the membership status of the potential defendant.
   C. Determines if allegation or inference constitutes a complaint of unethical conduct as defined in the *Principles of Medical Ethics with Annotations Especially Applicable to Psychiatry*—that is, does the allegation or inference merit an investigation—and, if so, files a copy of the complaint with the Secretary of the American Psychiatric Association.

II. Secretary of the American Psychiatric Association:
   A. Receives written and signed copy of the complaint from the District Branch and refers complaint back to the Branch for investigation.
   B. Notifies the accused member that a copy of a complaint has been received and filed, that the investigation will be conducted by the District Branch, and of the member's right to appeal a negative decision to the Board of Trustees of the American Psychiatric Association.

---

[3]Approved by the Executive Committee and the Assembly, 1975; revision approved by the Board of Trustees and the Assembly, 1977.

[4]Chapter 10, Section 1, By-Laws, American Psychiatric Association, 1981 revision.

III. District Branch:
- A. Upon receiving complaint from the secretary of the American Psychiatric Association, notifies the accused member of the complaint, who made the complaint, relates the complaint to the appropriate Section(s) of the *Principles of Medical Ethics with Annotations Especially Applicable to Psychiatry,* informs the accused member of his/her right to be advised and represented by legal counsel, and forwards to him/her a copy of the complaint, these Procedures, the *Principles of Medical Ethics with Annotations Especially Applicable to Psychiatry,* all addenda to the Procedures and Principles, and a copy of the Constitution and By-Laws of the American Psychiatric Association.
- B. Notifies complainant that the complaint has been received and will be investigated, of his/her right to legal counsel during the investigation, and that he/she will be informed of the decision of the District Branch.
- C. Refers the complaint to the District Branch Ethics Committee or whatever body serves that function for investigation and recommendations for action to the Council of the District Branch.
- D. Ethics Committee or whatever body serves that function investigates the complaint, permitting both the defendant and complainant to be heard. If the complainant is expected to produce evidence, he/she should be so advised in writing.
- E. May refer the complaint to the American Psychiatric Association for investigation under unusual circumstances and then Procedure B would be followed, with the APA Ethics Committee conducting the investigation. Unusual circumstances would include, but not be limited to, conflicts of interest, interested parties from different parts of the country, or a complaint of significant national importance.
- F. The Council of the District Branch, upon receiving the recommendation for action, determines:
  1. Either that the complaint is without merit and dismisses it.
  2. Or, that the complaint has been sustained and the defendant shall be subject to one of the following penalties:
     - a. Admonishment.
     - b. Reprimand.
     - c. Suspension from membership for a specific period of time.
     - d. Expulsion from the District Branch.
- G. Notifies the secretary of the American Psychiatric Association of the procedures followed, the Section under which the complaint was filed, and the action taken.

IV. Secretary of the American Psychiatric Association:
- A. Receives the report of the District Branch.
- B. Sends the report to the Ethics Committee of the American Psychiatric Association.

V. Ethics Committee of the American Psychiatric Association:
- A. Reviews the procedures followed by the District Branch.

B. Obtains additional information from the District Branch about procedures if necessary.

C. Reports to the Board of Trustees on the procedures followed and the action taken.

VI. Board of Trustees of the American Psychiatric Association:

A. On recommendation of the Ethics Committee of the American Psychiatric Association:

1. Approves that proper procedures have been followed. If not approved, the District Branch is directed to complete this investigation properly following the procedures.

2. Receives the report of action taken.

3. Orders the action taken be kept in a confidential file, listed by initial of the defendant only.

4. When expulsion from the District Branch is the action, notifies the defendant of his expulsion from the American Psychiatric Association and his right of appeal.

B. Instructs the secretary of the American Psychiatric Association to notify the District Branch whether or not proper procedures have been followed.

VII. District Branch:

A. Notifies the accused member of action taken and his/her rights of appeal.

B. Notifies complainant of action taken after avenues of appeal to the American Psychiatric Association have been exhausted or waived.

VIII. Appeal Procedure:

A. Within thirty (30) days of receipt of notice of action by the District Branch (and the Board of Trustees in case of expulsion), the defendant files written notice of his/her appeal with the secretary of the American Psychiatric Association.

B. The secretary of the American Psychiatric Association notifies the District Branch of the appeal and asks them to submit all information in their possession. The defendant is asked to submit the justification for his/her appeal and any information which he/she has which would support his/her appeal.

C. This information is submitted to the APA Ethics Committee. The defendant, with thirty (30) days' written notice, has the right to personal appearance, accompanied by legal counsel if he/she wishes, before the APA Ethics Committee. The APA Ethics Committee has the right to request the defendant and/or complainant to appear, with legal counsel if desired by either. (See Procedure B.IV.D.)

Procedure B. Allegation received by the American Psychiatric Association

I. Secretary of the American Psychiatric Association:

A. Receives signed communication alleging or inferring unethical conduct.

B. Determines the membership status of the potential defendant.

C. Determines if allegation or inference constitutes a complaint of unethical conduct as defined in the *Principles of Medical Ethics with Annotations Especially Applicable to Psychiatry*—that is, does the allegation or inference merit an investigation.

D. Notifies the accused member of the complaint, who made the complaint, relates the complaint to the appropriate Sections(s) of the *Principles of Medical Ethics with Annotations Especially Applicable to Psychiatry,* informs the accused member of his/her right to be advised and represented by legal counsel, and forwards to him/her a copy of the complaint, these Procedures, the *Principles of Medical Ethics with Annotations Especially Applicable to Psychiatry,* all addenda to the Procedures and Principles, and a copy of the Constitution and By-Laws of the American Psychiatric Association.

E. Notifies complainant that complaint has been received, that an investigation will be conducted by the District Branch (or APA Ethics Committee), advises him/her of his/her right to legal counsel during the investigation, and that he/she will be informed of the decison.

F. Sends complaint to the District Branch for investigation with information to the APA Ethics Committe.

II. District Branch:

A. Accepts the responsibility and assigns investigation to its Ethics Committee or whatever body acts in that capacity (and the Committee follows Procedure A.I); recommendations from that body are made to the Council of the District Branch.

B. The Council of the District Branch determines:

1. Either that the complaint is without merit and dismisses it.

2. Or, that the complaint has been sustained and the defendant shall be subject to one of the following penalties:

   a. Admonishment.

   b. Reprimand.

   c. Suspension from membership for a specific period of time.

   d. Expulsion from the District Branch.

C. The Council of the District Branch notifies the secretary of the American Psychiatric Association of the procedures followed and the action recommended.

III. Secretary of the American Psychiatric Association:

A. Reviews the procedures and recommendations of the District Branch.

B. Sends the report to the APA Ethics Committee.

IV. Ethics Committee of the American Psychiatric Association:

A. Reviews the procedures and recommendations of the District Branch.

B. Obtains additional information from the District Branch about procedures and recommendations if necessary.

C. Reports to the APA Board of Trustees on the procedures followed and actions recommended.

D. When the APA Ethics Committee is the original investigating body:

1. The Ethics Committee may request two Fellows of the American Psychiatric Association residing in the same area as the complainant and defendant to serve as investigators. These investigators may interview the parties and gather other pertinent information, which they will submit to the Ethics Committee. If the complainant is expected to produce evidence, he/she should be so advised in writing.

2. Because of possible distances involved, the defendant and complainant

shall be given thirty (30) day's notice in writing of the time and place of the meeting of the Ethics Committee.

3. The defendant and complainant shall have the right to appear and to legal counsel.
4. The Ethics Committee makes its recommendation to the Board of Trustees.

V. Board of Trustees of the American Psychiatric Association:
   A. On recommendation of the APA Ethics Committee:
      1. Approves that proper procedures have been followed. If not approved, the District Branch (or the Ethics Committee if the investigating body) is directed to complete their investigation properly following the procedures.
      2. Approves, disapproves, or modifies the action recommended by the District Branch (or the Ethics Committee if the investigating body). In case of expulsion, a two-thirds (⅔) vote of the Board of Trustees is required.
      3. Notifies the complainant after avenues of appeal have been exhausted or waived, and the defendant and the District Branch of the action taken. The defendant is again advised of his/her right to appeal and to be represented by legal counsel.
      4. Orders the action taken be kept in a confidential file, listed by initial of the defendant only.
      5. In the case of expulsion, the member is also expelled from the District Branch.

VI. Appeal Procedure:
   A. Within thirty (30) days of receipt of notice of action by the APA Board of Trustees, the defendant files written notice with the secretary of the American Psychiatric Association of his/her appeal.
   B. Expelled members shall be denied all membership privileges pending the appeal.
   C. All other penalties shall be suspended pending the appeal.
   D. The appeal shall be heard at the next Annual Meeting of the American Psychiatric Association at a session attended only by voting members and the necessary secretarial staff and legal counsel as selected by the president.
   E. The defendant shall have the right to be heard, present his/her evidence, and be represented by legal counsel.
   F. Presentation of evidence and arguments for the American Psychiatric Association shall be made by the president or a member of his choice.
   G. A two-thirds (⅔) vote of those present by secret written ballot shall be required to reverse the action of the Board of Trustees, leading to a modified action or dismissal of the charges.

OUTLINE OF DISTRICT BRANCH REPORT TO THE AMERICAN PSYCHIATRIC ASSOCIATION (AFTER INVESTIGATION)

Dear Secretary:

We have concluded our investigation into the ethical complaint filed against Dr. _____ about which we previously notified you on _____. The following procedures were followed:

	Yes	*No*

1. The accused member was interviewed by our ethics committe or other investigating body.
2. The accused member was represented by counsel.
3. The accused member called witnesses on his/her behalf.
4. The accused member introduced other evidence on his/her behalf.
5. The complainant or his/her legal counsel questioned the accused member and/or other witnesses.
6. The complainant was interviewed by our ethics committee or other investigating body.
7. The complainant was represented by counsel.
8. The complainant called witnesses on his/her behalf.
9. The complainant introduced other evidence on his/her behalf.
10. The accused member and/or his/her counsel questioned the complainant and other witnesses.

Describe any other procedures followed: _____
_____
_____

On the basis of our investigation, we have found the accused member in violation of the Principles of Medical Ethics with Annotations Especially Applicable to Psychiatry, Section _____. Our basis for this conclusion is as follows:

(Here the District Branch should include a brief statement—½ to 1 page—of the reasons for its decision; e.g., accused member admitted, complainant's allegations did not withstand questioning, documentary evidence, etc.)

We believe that the accused member should be (admonished, reprimanded, suspended [for _____ years], expelled). Our basis for this sanction is as follows:

(Here the District Branch should give a brief statement—¼ to ½ page—of its reasons for the sanction; e.g., very serious offense, accused member in treatment, not likely to repeat, etc.)

SUGGESTED DISTRICT BRANCH LETTER TO THE ACCUSED MEMBER (BEFORE INVESTIGATION)

Dear Dr. _____:

This is to notify you that an ethical complaint against you has been filed by _____. A copy of the complaint is enclosed. The complaint alleges violations of the Principles of Medical Ethics with Annotations Especially Applicable to Psychiatry, Section _____. This district branch will be investigating the complaint. You are advised that you have the right to be represented by legal counsel during these proceedings. We will notify you as the investigation proceeds.

We are enclosing a copy of the Constitution and By-Laws of the American Psychiatric Association, as well as a copy of the Procedures for Handling Complaints of Unethical Conduct and the Principles of Medical Ethics with Annotations Especially Applicable to Psychiatry.

If you have any questions, please write to this district branch.

Very truly yours,

E. American Dental Association Principles of Ethics and Code of Professional Conduct*

The maintenance and enrichment of professional status place on everyone who practices dentistry an obligation which should be willingly accepted and willingly fulfilled. While the basic obligation is constant, its fulfillment may vary with the changing needs of a society composed of the human beings that a profession is dedicated to serve. The spirit of the obligation, therefore, must be the guide of conduct for professionals. This obligation has been summarized for all time in the golden rule which asks only that "whatsoever ye would that men should do to you, do ye even so to them."

The practice of dentistry first achieved the stature of a profession in the United States when, through the heritage bestowed by the efforts of many generations of dentists, it acquired the three unfailing characteristics of a profession: the primary duty of service to the public, education beyond the usual level, and the responsibility for self-government.

PRINCIPLE—SECTION 1

Service to the public and quality of care

The dentist's primary obligation of service to the public shall include the delivery of quality care, competently and timely, within the bounds of the clinical circumstances presented by the patient. Quality of care shall be a primary consideration of the dental practitioner.

CODE OF PROFESSIONAL CONDUCT

1–A. **Patient selection.** While dentists, in serving the public, any exercise reasonable discretion in selecting patients for their practices, dentists shall not refuse to accept

---

*Principles of Ethics and Code of Professional Conduct, (with official advisory opinions) ADA, July 1982. Reprinted with permission from the American Dental Association, Council on Bylaws and Judicial Affairs.

181

patients into their practice or deny dental service to patients because of the patient's race, creed, color, sex or national origin.

1–B. Patient records. Dentists are obliged to safeguard the confidentiality of patient records. Dentists shall maintain patient records in a manner consistent with the protection of the welfare of the patient. Upon request of a patient or another dental practitioner, dentists shall provide any information that will be beneficial for the future treatment of that patient.

ADVISORY OPINION

1. A dentist has the ethical obligation on request of either the patient or the patient's new dentist to furnish, either gratuitously or for nominal cost, such dental records or copies or summaries of them, including dental x-rays or copies of them, as will be beneficial for the future treatment of that patient.

1–C. Community service. Since dentists have an obligation to use their skills, knowledge, and experience for the improvement of the dental health of the public and are encouraged to be leaders in their community, dentists in such service shall conduct themselves in such a manner as to maintain or elevate the esteem of the profession.

1–D. Emergency service. Dentists shall be obliged to make reasonable arrangements for the emergency care of their patients of record.

Dentists shall be obliged when consulted in an emergency by patients not of record to make reasonable arrangements for emergency care. If treatment is provided, the dentist, upon completion of such treatment, is obliged to return the patient to his or her regular dentist unless the patient expressly reveals a different preference.

1–E. Consultation and referral. Dentists shall be obliged to seek consultation, if possible, whenever the welfare of patients will be safeguarded or advanced by utilizing those who have special skills, knowledge and experience. When patients visit or are referred to specialists or consulting dentists for consultation:

1. The specialists or consulting dentists upon completion of their care shall return the patient, unless the patient expressly reveals a different preference, to the referring dentist, or if none, to the dentist of record for future care.

2. The specialists shall be obliged when there is no referring dentist and upon a completion of their treatment to inform patients when there is a need for further dental care.

1–F. Use of auxiliary personnel. Dentists shall be obliged to protect the health of their patient by only assigning to qualified auxiliaries those duties which can be legally delegated. Dentists shall be further obliged to prescribe and supervise the work of all auxiliary personnel working under their direction and control.

1–G. Justifiable criticism. Dentists shall be obliged to report to the appropriate reviewing agency as determined by the local component or constituent society instances of gross and continual faulty treatment by other dentists. Patients should be informed of their present oral health status without disparaging comment about prior services.

1–H. Expert testimony. Dentists may provide expert testimony when that testimony is essential to a just and fair disposition of a judicial or administrative action.

1–I. Rebate and split fees. Dentists shall not accept or tender "rebates" or "split fees."

1–J. Representation of care and fees. Dentists shall not represent the care being rendered to their patients or the fees being charged for providing such care in a false or misleading manner.

ADVISORY OPINIONS

1. A dentist who accepts a third-party[1] payment under a copayment plan as payment in full without disclosing to the third-party payer that the patient's payment portion will not be collected, is engaged in overbilling. The essence of this ethical impropriety is deception and misrepresentation; an overbilling dentist makes it appear to the third-party payer that the charge to the patient for services rendered is higher than it actually is.

2. It is unethical for a dentist to increase a fee to a patient solely because the patient has insurance.

3. Payments accepted by a dentist under a governmentally funded program, a component or constituent dental society sponsored access program or a participating agreement entered into under a program of a third party shall not be considered as evidence of overbilling in determining whether a charge to a patient, or to another third party in behalf of a patient not covered under any of the afore cited programs constitutes overbilling under this section of the *Code*.

4. A dentist who submits a claim form to a third party reporting incorrect treatment dates for the purpose of assisting a patient in obtaining benefits under a dental plan, which benefits would otherwise be disallowed, is engaged in making an unethical, false, and misleading representation to such third party.

5. A dentist who incorrectly describes on a third-party claim form a dental procedure in order to receive a greater payment or reimbursement or incorrectly makes a noncovered procedure appear to be a covered procedure on such a claim from is engaged in making an unethical, false, and misleading representation to such third party.

6. A dentist who recommends and performs unnecessary dental services or procedures is engaged in unethical conduct.

PRINCIPLE—SECTION 2

Education

The privilege of dentists to be accorded professional status rests primarily in the knowledge, skill and experience with which they serve their patients and society. All dentists, therefore, have the obligation of keeping their knowledge and skill current.

PRINCIPLE—SECTION 3

Government of a profession

Every profession owes society the responsibility to regulate itself. Such regulation is achieved largely through the influence of the professional societies. All dentists, there-

---

[1]A third party is any party to a dental prepayment contract that may collect premiums, assume financial risks, pay claims, and/or provide administrative services.

fore, have the dual obligation of making themselves a part of a professional society and of observing its rules of ethics.

PRINCIPLE—SECTION 4

Research and development

Dentists have the obligation of making the results and benefits of their investigative efforts available to all when they are useful in safeguarding or promoting the health of the public.

CODE OF PROFESSIONAL CONDUCT

4–A. Devices and therapeutic methods. Except for formal investigative studies, dentists shall be obliged to prescribe, dispense, or promote only those devices, drugs, and other agents whose complete formulae are available to the dental profession. Dentists shall have the further obligation of not holding out as exclusive any device, agent, method or technique.

4–B. Patents and copyrights. Patents and copyrights may be secured by dentists provided that such patents and copyrights shall not be used to restrict research or practice.

PRINCIPLE—SECTION 5

Professional announcement

In order to properly serve the public, dentists should represent themselves in a manner that contributes to the esteem of the profession. Dentists should not misrepresent their training and competence in any way that would be false or misleading in any material respect.[2]

CODE OF PROFESSIONAL CONDUCT

5–A. Advertising. Although any dentist may advertise, no dentist shall advertise or solicit patients in any form of communication in a manner that is false or misleading in any material respect.

ADVISORY OPINION

1. If a dental health article, message, or newsletter is published under a dentist's byline to the public without making truthful disclosure of the source and authorship or is designed to give rise to questionable expectations for the purpose of inducing the public

---

[2]Advertising, solicitation of patients or business, or other promotional activities by dentists or dental care delivery organizations shall not be considered unethical or improper, except for those promotional activities which are false or misleading in any material respect. Notwithstanding any ADA *Principles of Ethics and Code of Professional Conduct* or other standards of dentist conduct which may be differently worded, this shall be the sole standard for determining the ethical propriety of such promotional activities. Any provision of an ADA constituent or component society's

to utilize the services of the sponsoring dentist, the dentist is engaged in making a false or misleading representation to the public in a material respect.

5–B. Name of practice. Since the name under which a dentist conducts his practice may be a factor in the selection process of the patient, the use of a trade name or an assumed name that is false or misleading in any material respect is unethical.

Use of the name of a dentist no longer actively associated with the practice may be continued for a period not to exceed one year.

5–C. Announcement of specialization and limitation of practice. This Section and Section 5–D are designed to help the public make an informed selection between the practitioner who has completed an accredited program beyond the dental degree and a practitioner who has not completed such a program.

The special areas of dental practice approved by the American Dental Association and the designation for ethical specialty announcement and limitation of practice are: dental public health, endodontics, oral pathology, oral and maxillofacial surgery, orthodontics, pedodontics (dentistry for children), periodontics and prosthodontics.

Dentists who choose to announce specialization should use "specialist in" or "practice limited to" and shall limit their practice exclusively to the announced special area(s) of dental practice, provided at the time of the announcement such dentists have met in each approved specialty for which they announce the existing educational requirements and standards set forth by the American Dental Association.

Dentists who use their eligibility to announce as specialists to make the public believe that specialty services rendered in the dental office are being rendered by qualified specialists when such is not the case are engaged in unethical conduct. The burden of responsibility is on specialists to avoid any inference that general practitioners who are associated with specialists are qualified to announce themselves as specialists.

General standards

The following are included within the standards of the American Dental Association for determining what dentists have the education, experience, and other appropriate requirements for announcing specialization and limitation of practice:

1. The special area(s) of dental practice and an appropriate certifying board must be approved by the American Dental Association.

2. Dentists who announce as specialists must have successfully completed an educational program accredited by the Commission on Dental Accreditation, two or more years in length, as specified by the Council on Dental Education or be diplomates of a nationally recognized certifying board.

3. The practice carried on by dentists who announce as specialists shall be limited exclusively to the special area(s) of dental practice announced by the dentist.

Standards for multiple-specialty announcements

Educational criteria for announcement by dentists in additional recognized specialty areas are the successful completion of an educational program accredited by the Commission on Dental Accreditation in each area for which the dentist wishes to announce.

code of ethics or other standard of dentist conduct relating to dentists' or dental care delivery organizations' advertising, solicitation, or other promotional activities which is worded differently from the above standard shall be deemed to be in conflict with the ADA *Principles of Ethics and Code of Professional Conduct.*

Dentists who completed their advanced education in programs listed by the Council in Dental Education prior to the initiation of the accreditation process in 1967 and who are currently ethically announcing as specialists in a recognized area may announce in additional areas provided they are educationally qualified or are certified diplomates in each area for which they wish to announce. Documentation of successful completion of the educational program(s) must be submitted to the appropriate constituent society. The documentation must assure that the duration of the program(s) is a minimum of two years except for oral and maxillofacial surgery which must have been a minimum of three years in duration.

5–D. General practitioner announcement of services. General dentists who wish to announce the services available in their practices are permitted to announce the availability of those services so long as they avoid any communications that express or imply specialization. General dentists shall also state that the services are being provided by general dentists. No dentists shall announce available services in any way that would be false or misleading in any material respect.

INTERPRETATION AND APPLICATION OF "PRINCIPLES OF ETHICS AND CODE OF PROFESSIONAL CONDUCT"

The preceding statements constitute the *Principles of Ethics and Code of Professional Conduct* of the American Dental Association. The purpose of the *Principles and Code* is to uphold and strengthen dentistry as a member of the learned professions. The constituent and component societies may adopt additional provisions or interpretations not in conflict with these *Principles of Ethics and Code of Professional Conduct* which would enable them to serve more faithfully the traditions, customs, and desires of the members of these societies.

Problems involving questions of ethics should be solved at the local level within the broad boundaries established in these *Principles of Ethics and Code of Professional Conduct* and within the interpretation by the component and/or constituent society of their respective codes of ethics. If a satisfactory decision cannot be reached, the question should be referred on appeal to the constituent society and the Council on Bylaws and Judicial Affairs of the American Dental Association, as provided in Chapter XI of the *Bylaws* of the American Dental Association. Members found guilty of unethical conduct as prescribed in the American Dental Association *Code of Professional Conduct* or codes of ethics of the constituent and component societies are subject to the penalties set forth in Chapter XI of the American Dental Association *Bylaws*.

APPENDIX II

Licensure laws and annotations for dentistry and psychology

A. Licensure for dentistry*

Educational requirements

Graduates of U.S. dental schools. Graduates of U.S. dental schools accredited by the ADA Commission on Accreditation are eligible for dental licensure in all U.S. jurisdictions.

Graduates of Canadian dental schools. Graduates of Canadian dental schools accredited by the ADA Commission on Accreditation are eligible for regular dental licensure in all U.S. jurisdictions *except* Alaska and Mississippi.

Graduates of foreign dental schools. Graduates of dental schools located outside of the United States and Canada may be eligible for dental licensure in Arizona, California, District of Columbia, Florida, Illinois, Maryland,[1] Massachusetts, Michigan, Minnesota, New York, Rhode Island, Tennessee, Texas, Utah, Washington, and Wisconsin. Specific licensure requirements for foreign dental graduates vary widely among the jurisdictions.

Licensure examinations

National Board examinations. All U.S. jurisdictions except Alabama and Delaware accept satisfactory scores on the National Board dental examination as fulfilling or partially fulfilling the state written examination requirement for licensure. In Missouri, candidates must have an average score of 75 with no more than two scores below 75 and none below 65.

Arizona and Hawaii have 5-year time limits for accepting National Board dental results. Puerto Rico, Florida, and Kansas have a 10-year time limit and Colorado has a 15-year time limit. Florida will have a 10-year time limit for accepting National Board dental results beginning July 1, 1979.

Dental candidates who have passed National Board dental examinations are required

---

*This information was compiled from a survey of state boards of dentistry jointly conducted by the American Association of Dental Examiners and the American Dental Association in late 1978/early 1979. The information concerning New Hampshire is from a survey conducted in late 1977. Current information for New Hampshire is not available at the present time. For more information on licensure requirements, please contact the appropriate state board of dentistry.

[1]Maryland requires that graduates of foreign dental schools who apply for licensure after November 17, 1978 attend a U.S. accredited dental school for two years.

188

to take additional written tests in all jurisdictions *except* Illinois, Iowa, Massachusetts, New York, and Rhode Island. These written tests vary among the jurisdictions.

State written examinations. Alabama and Delaware accept only satisfactory scores on their respective state written examinations as fulfilling their written examination requirements for licensure. Jurisdictions that offer their own written examinations in addition to accepting National Board results are Arizona, Arkansas, Colorado, District of Columbia, Hawaii, Idaho, Indiana, Mississippi, Nebraska, Nevada, Oklahoma, Oregon, Puerto Rico, and Virginia. Virginia's written examination is available only to dentists who graduated prior to July 1, 1966. Missouri's written examination is available only to dentists who graduated prior to January 1, 1965.

Examination sequencing. Jurisdictions which allow a candidate for licensure to take the clinical examination *before* he has fulfilled written examination requirements are Arizona, Arkansas, Colorado, Connecticut, Florida, Kansas, Massachusetts, Minnesota, Mississippi, New Hampshire, New Jersey, New York, Ohio, Oklahoma, Utah, Vermont, Virginia, and Wisconsin.

Regional testing. Following are the 34 jurisdictions that participate in regional clinical testing services for dentistry. Time limits for accepting regional testing service results are listed in parentheses.

Central Regional Dental Testing Service—Colorado (5 yrs.), Iowa (5 yrs.), Kansas (5 yrs.), Minnesota (5 yrs.), Missouri (5 yrs.), Nebraska (5 yrs.), North Dakota (5 yrs.), Oklahoma (5 yrs.), South Dakota (5 yrs.), Wisconsin (5 yrs.), and Wyoming (5 yrs.). Under certain circumstances, Wisconsin also recognizes Northeast Regional Board results. The state of Wisconsin Board of Dentistry should be contacted for exact information.

Northeast Regional Board—Connecticut (5 yrs.), District of Columbia (5 yrs.), Illinois (5 yrs.), Maine (5 yrs.), Maryland (5 yrs.), Massachusetts (5 yrs.), Michigan (5 yrs.), New Hampshire (5 yrs.), New Jersey (10 yrs.), New York (10 yrs.), Ohio (5 yrs.), Pennsylvania (5 yrs.), Rhode Island (none), Vermont (5 yrs.), and West Virginia (5 yrs.). Michigan recognizes CRDTS results on an individual basis.

Southern Regional Testing Agency—Arkansas (5 yrs.), Kentucky (5 yrs.), Tennessee (5 yrs.), and Virginia (5 yrs.).

Western Regional Examining Board—Arizona (5 yrs.). Montana[2] (3 yrs.), Oregon (3 yrs.), and Utah (3 yrs.).

A state performance examination is available for dental candidates who have not passed the regional dental examination in the following jurisdictions: Arizona, Connecticut, District of Columbia, Illinois, Maryland, Massachusetts, Nebraska, New York, and Tennessee.

Alternate mechanisms of licensure

Licensure by credentials. Licensure by credentials is the licensing of a dentist previously licensed in another state without examination on the basis of his credentials meeting specific professional criteria established by the state board of dentistry. Jurisdic-

---

[2]Montana will participate beginning in June 1979.

tions offering licensure by credentials for dentistry are Indiana, Kansas, Maine, Maryland, Massachusetts, Minnesota, Missouri, Nebraska, New York, Ohio, Oklahoma, Pennsylvania, Rhode Island, South Dakota, Tennessee, and Wyoming.

In the following jurisdictions, dentists licensed by credentials are required to pass a portion of the dental licensure examination battery used by the jurisdiction: Indiana, Kansas, Maine, Maryland, Minnesota, Missouri, Pennsylvania, South Dakota, and Tennessee. The specific requirement varies among jurisdictions.

Graduates of ADA recognized Canadian dental schools, previously licensed only in Canadian provinces, are eligible for licensure by credentials in the following jurisdictions: Indiana, Maine, Maryland, Minnesota, Missouri, Ohio, Pennsylvania, South Dakota, and Wyoming. In New York, graduates of Canadian dental schools are eligible for licensure by credentials only if able to provide proof of an equivalent examination.

License recognition. Table IIA-1 indicates jurisdictions that recognize dental licenses issued by specific jurisdictions.

TABLE IIA-1

Jurisdiction	Recognizes licenses issued by:
Illinois	Indiana, Iowa, Massachusetts, New Jersey, North Dakota, Pennsylvania, Rhode Island, and West Virginia.
New Jersey	Illinois and Pennsylvania.
South Dakota	CRDTS states
Puerto Rico	Illinois and Ohio

Temporary licenses. Alaska, Hawaii, Idaho, Louisiana, Michigan, North Carolina, and West Virginia have provision for issuing temporary licenses to dentists who move into the state so they can practice while awaiting examination for regular licenses.

The following jurisdictions provide for issuing temporary licenses to dentists who have arranged to volunteer their services for a short period of time with a recognized charitable organization working in disadvantaged or remote rural areas: Arizona (restricted permit), Florida, Hawaii, Louisiana, Maine, Michigan, Mississippi, New Mexico, North Carolina, Puerto Rico, and Tennessee.

Specialty licenses. Jurisdictions conducting specialty licensure are Alaska, Arkansas, District of Columbia, Kansas, Kentucky, Michigan, Mississippi, Missouri, Nevada, Oklahoma, Oregon, South Carolina, Tennessee, and West Virginia. Table IIA-2 indicates the specialties licensed by each jurisdiction.

Provisional licenses. The following jurisdictions have provision for issuing provisional licenses to full-time school faculty members to allow them to discharge faculty duties: Alabama, California, Colorado, Connecticut, Florida ("teaching permits"), Georgia, Indiana, Iowa, Kentucky ("courtesy license"), Louisiana ("restricted license"), Maryland, Massachusetts, Michigan, Mississippi, Nevada, New Jersey, New York ("limited permit"), North Dakota, Ohio ("teaching certificate"), Oklahoma, Puerto Rico, Tennessee, Virginia, and West Virginia ("teaching permit").

In Arizona, Arkansas, South Carolina, and Texas, full-time faculty members are exempted from dental licensure as long as they do not engage in private practice.

TABLE IIA-2

	Dental Public Health	Endo- dontics	Oral Pa- thology	Oral and Maxillo- facial Surgery	Ortho- dontics	Pedo- dontics	Perio- dontics	Prostho dontics
Alaska								
Arkansas	—	X	—	X	X	X	X	X
District of Columbia	—	X	X	X	X	X	X	—
Kansas	X	X	—	X	X	X	X	X
Kentucky								
Michigan	—	X	—	X	X	X	X	X
Mississippi								
Missouri	X	X	X	X	X	X	X	X
Nevada								
Oklahoma	—	X	X	X	X	X	X	X
Oregon	—	X	X	X	X	X	X	X
South Carolina								
Tennessee								
West Virginia	X	X	X	X(A)	X	X	X	X

Blanks indicate the information was not available for this survey.
(A) Oral Surgery only.
The specific requirements necessary to obtain a specialty license vary among the jurisdictions. The State Boards of Dentistry should be contacted for exact information.

In West Virginia, the "teaching permit" must be followed by a permanent license within a year.

Residency requirements. Delaware requires one year of general practice residency or its equivalent for licensure. Puerto Rico has a 6-month residency requirement.

Licensure maintenance

Continuing education. Table IIA-3 shows state education requirements for licensure renewal. In addition to the jurisdictions listed, Puerto Rico is in the process of establishing a continuing education requirement.

TABLE IIA-3

Arizona (effective 7/1/79)	N/A
California	50 credit hours every 2 years
Iowa	N/A
Kansas	30 credit hours per year
Kentucky	10 points per year
Minnesota	75 credit hours every 5 years
New Mexico	60 credit hours every 3 years
North Dakota	50 credit hours every 5 years
Oklahoma	20 credit hours per year
Oregon	40 credit hours every 3 years
South Dakota	75 credit hours every 5 years

Inactive status. In Connecticut, Idaho, Iowa, Mississippi, New Jersey, Oregon, and South Dakota, dentists licensed in the state, but residing and/or practicing outside the state can be placed on inactive status. In Nebraska, Nevada, New York, North Carolina, Ohio, and Pennsylvania, licensed dentists are placed on inactive status only upon request.

TABLE IIA–4

	Initial fee for dental licensure	Reregistration fee for dental licensure	
Alabama	$ 60	$ 10	Annually
Alaska	30	40	Biennially
Arizona	125	35	Annually
Arkansas	75	40	Annually
California	150	60	Biennially
Colorado	114	22.75	Biennially
Connecticut	150	150	Annually
Delaware	75	20	Biennially
District of Columbia	(A)	20	Annually
Florida	125	70	Biennially
Georgia	74	40	Biennially
Hawaii	60	21	Biennially
Idaho	55	55	Annually
Illinois	50	10	Biennially
Indiana	50	60	Biennially
Iowa	50	15	Annually
Kansas	50	25	Annually
Kentucky	50	25	Annually
Louisiana	50	30	Annually
Maine	50	20	Biennially
Maryland	50	5	Annually
Massachusetts	75	30	Biennially
Michigan	35	25	Annually
Minnesota (C)	70	38	Annually
Mississippi	100	50	Annually
Missouri	60	15	Annually
Montana	65	25	Annually
Nebraska	50	15	Annually
Nevada	100	50	Biennially
New Hampshire	150	50	Biennially
New Jersey	50	50	Biennially
New Mexico	150	15	Annually
New York	(B)	40	Biennially
North Carolina	75	40	Annually
North Dakota	75	40	Annually
Ohio	30	30	Annually
Oklahoma	60	40	Annually
Oregon	50	50	Annually
Pennsylvania (D)	25	25	Biennially
Puerto Rico	25	–	Biennially
Rhode Island	75	25	Annually
South Carolina	150	25	Annually
South Dakota	50	35	Annually
Tennessee	50	20	Annually
Texas	100	50	Annually
Utah	20	10	Annually

TABLE IIA–4 *(concluded)*

	Initial fee for dental licensure	Reregistration fee for dental licensure	
Vermont	50	25	Annually
Virginia	100	40	Biennially
Washington	50	15	Annually
West Virginia	35	20	Annually
Wisconsin	50	30	Biennially
Wyoming	100	35	Annually

(A) $30 if based examination on District of Columbia examination; $40 if based on Northeast Regional Board examination.
(B) $140 if state examination is required; $100 if state examination is not required.
(C) $250 by credentials.
(D) $50 by credentials.

B. Licensure for Psychology*

THE PURPOSE OF LICENSURE OR CERTIFICATION OF PSYCHOLOGISTS[1]

The practice of professional psychology is now regulated by law in 49 of the 50 states of the United States, as well as the District of Columbia and 7 provinces of Canada.[2] The laws are intended to protect the public by limiting licensure to those persons who are qualifed to practice psychology as defined by state law.

The legal basis for licensure lies in the right of the state to enact legislation to protect its citizens. *Caveat emptor* or "buyer beware," is felt to be an unsound maxim when the "buyer" of services cannot be sufficiently well informed to beware, and hence states have established regulatory boards to license qualified practitioners. A professional board is a state agency acting to protect the public, not to serve the profession. However, by insuring high standards for those who practice independently, the board is simultaneously serving the best interests of both the public and profession. The major functions of any professional board are: (1) to determine the standards for admission into the profession and to administer appropriate procedures for selection and examination and (2) to regulate practice and to conduct disciplinary proceedings involving violation of standards of professional conduct embodied in law.

Those who practice the profession of psychology in a research laboratory, in a state or federal institution or agency, or in a college or university are still exempt from the requirements of licensure in some states, although there is a trend toward requiring licensure of agency employees. The psychologist who offers direct services to the public for a fee must be licensed.

TYPICAL REQUIREMENTS OF PSYCHOLOGY LICENSING LAWS

Licensing laws in the various jurisdictions differ considerably, yet most have a common core of agreement. Of course, each board is the final authority on all matters of

---

*Reprinted from *Entry Requirements for Professional Practice of Psychology: A Guide for Students and Faculty,* (New York: American Association of State Psychology Boards).

[1]When both the title and practice of psychology are regulated, the law is called a *licensing* law; when only the title of psychologist is regulated, the law is called a *certification* law: To avoid redundancy in the remainder of our discussion the word "licensure" will be used to stand for either licensure or certification.

[2]Throughout this text the term "state" will refer to Canada's provinces as well as political subdivisions of the United States.

requirements within its jurisdiction and should be contacted for specifics. The typical requirements for licensure in the various jurisdictions are as follows:

A. *Education.* Achievement of a doctoral degree in psychology from an approved program, or the equivalent as deemed by the board. The definitions of approved programs vary widely, but often refer to accreditation of the academic institutions by recognized accrediting bodies. (Some states have two or more levels of licensure or certification, with the lower level requiring less than the doctoral degree and entailing more restrictions on the practitioner.)

B. *Experience.* One or two years supervised experience in a setting approved by the state board. Most, but not all, states require that some of the supervised experience be postdoctoral.

C. *Examination.* Demonstration of relevant knowledge through passing an objective written examination. The Examination of Professional Practice in Psychology, constructed by a committee of AASPB in association with the Professional Examination Service, is used in about 48 jurisdictions. The cut-off point for successful performance on the examination is determined by the board having authority for the jurisdiction. In some states, successful performance is required on an oral and/or essay examination conducted by the board or a committee designated by the board. Specialty examinations, e.g., in clinical psychology, industrial psychology, or school psychology may become common in the near future.

D. *Administrative requirements.* In addition to the foregoing requirements, the various state laws specify different citizenship, age, and residence requirements, as well as requiring evidence of good moral character.

Stated succinctly, the major hurdles which any candidate must meet in the evaluation by the board are:

1. The boards's review of credentials (transcripts, application, references).
2. Examination (written and/or oral)

Most candidates successfully pass these hurdles, but some fail. Potential sources of difficulty are discussed below.

HOW TO PREPARE FOR SUCCESSFULLY MEETING THE REQUIREMENTS OF LICENSURE

Although well prepared candidates have little or no problem with the licensing process, certain areas can be identified in which difficulties are most likely to occur. These potential problem areas are:

1. Knowledge of the law and regulations. The applicant should examine the law for the jurisdiction in which licensure is sought to assure that there has been full compliance with the law before an application is submitted. The applicant also should be familiar with, and comply with, any regulations of the board with respect to qualifications.

2. Adequacy of training and/or experience. The problems subsumed under this heading include a lack of the appropriate degree specified by the law (usually a Ph.D. in psychology); failure of the candidate to complete the required number of graduate hours in psychology; failure of the institution from which the degree was granted to meet the criteria for approval by the board; failure of the specific curriculum in which the student was enrolled to meet the requirements of the particular state board. With regard to the last-mentioned criterion, most laws contain a stipulation that the graduate work be predominantly psychological in nature, and the doctoral degree be based upon a dissertation which is psychological in content. It should also be noted that some jurisdictions require evidence of continuing education, beyond the Ph.D., for psychologists to retain their licenses.

In addition to these problems having to do with the nature of the candidate's education, each law specifies the duration of experience required, and each board stipulates the type of setting in which approved experience may be obtained. Typical of such approved settings are the APA-approved internship programs. Each candidate should plan for supervised experience that will satisfy the legal requirements for practice in the jurisdiction in which licensure is desired.

3. Examination performance. Successful performance in state licensing examinations usually requires demonstration of knowledge of basic psychology which is relevant to professional practice, along with knowledge of professional ethics and professional affairs. While numerous factors are undoubtedly operative, probably the most frequent source of failure is the candidate's possession of insufficient knowledge of basic psychology. Candidates may also be disqualified in oral examinations as a consequence of demonstration of insufficient knowledge about the management of professional problems, particularly ethical problems.

THE CONTENT OF EXAMINATION OF PROFESSIONAL PRACTICE IN PSYCHOLOGY

In order to help the candidate to prepare for the Examination of Professional Practice in Psychology (EPPP), a separate brochure has been prepared by AASPB, and is available from AASPB, the Professional Examination Service, or the board of examiners in those jurisdictions using the exam. In the paragraphs below, the content of that examination is summarized briefly.

1. Background knowledge: physiological psychology and comparative psychology, learning, history, theory and systems, sensation and perception, motivation, social-psychology, personality, cognitive processes, developmental psychology, psychopharmacology.
2. Methodology: research design and interpretation, statistics, test construction and interpretation, scaling.
3. Professional practice:
   a. Clinical psychology: test usage and interpretation, diagnoses, psychopathology, therapy, judgment in clinical situations, community health.
   b. Behavior modification: learning, applications.
   c. Other specialities: management consulting, industrial and human engineering, social psychology, T-groups, counseling and guidance, communications, systems analysis.
   d. Professional conduct, affairs, and ethics: interdisciplinary relations, professional conduct, knowledge of professional affairs.

The EPPP is published in various forms, with new forms published periodically. The examination varies from 150 to 200 items in length. The content areas enumerated above are not equally weighted.

The requirements for licensure, delineated above, and the discussion of potential bases for denial, suggest that the student who seeks out a broad and sophisticated background in psychology is likely to encounter few problems in the licensing process. The student should especially seek experiences which emphasize the application of psychological knowledge to problems likely to be encountered as a professional psychologist. Narrowly based training, avoiding the complexity of the field of psychology, is probably not in the student's best interest if professional practice is a goal. Cursory or limited supervision, or supervision by other than a qualified psychologist, is also likely to lead to deficiencies. Moreover, since psychologists tend to be mobile, a broad background acceptable to all or most boards is preferable to training narrowly designed to meet the requirements of a single jurisdiction. Students who have sought out experiences consistent with APA standards and have taken training at recognized facilities of quality rarely experience difficulty in obtaining licensure.

An Interstate Reporting Service has been established by the Professional Examination Service to facilitate mobility by permitting easier endorsement of licenses among states. The Reporting Service maintains a permanent record of examination scores on the EPPP for those candidates who choose to register. On the candidate's request, the Service will report the score, accompanied by appropriate normative data, to the board of another state in which licensure is being sought.

RESOURCES

It cannot be overemphasized that the final and absolute word concerning requirements for licensure in any state must be obtained from the specific board in question. Addresses for state boards are published each calendar year in the *American Psychologist*. When in doubt, write or call your board. In addition to the individual boards, the following are other sources of information which may be of value to students and faculty.

American Association of State Psychology Boards
c/o Morton Berger, Ph.D.
N.Y. State Board of Psychology
99 Washington Avenue, Rm. 1841
Albany, New York 12230

American Psychological Association
Office of Professional Affairs
1200 Seventeenth Street, N.W.
Washington, D.C. 20036

American Psychological Association
Office of Educational Affairs
1200 Seventeenth Street, N.W.
Washington, D.C. 20036

Standards for Providers of Psychological Services.
American Psychological Association, September 1974.

Certification and licensure

State and provincial laws regulating psychological practice are usually either Licensure (L) or Certification (C) laws. Certification regulates the use of the title "psycholo-

CHART 1

A summary of laws regulating the practice of psychology through (L) Licensure or (C) Certification

State		First approved in	Major amendments	Coverage	Educational requirements	Post degree	Supervision	Total experience	ABPP recognized	Mandatory examination	Continuing education for renewal	Renewal every	Psychology members	Public members	Terms	"Grandparenting" ends
													Examining board			
Alabama	(L)	1963		Practice of Psychologists	Doctorate	—	—	0	yes	yes	no	1 yr.	5	—	5	10/1/65
Alaska	(L)	1967		Psychologist	Doctorate	1	1	1	yes	yes	yes	4 yrs.	3	2	2	1/1/68
Arizona	(C)	1965	1978	Psychological Associate	Masters	1	3	3	—	yes	no	4 yrs.	5	2	5	1974
Arkansas	(L)	1955		Psychologist	Doctorate	—	—	0	yes	yes	yes	1 yr.	5	1	5	7/1/57
California	(L)	1957		Psychological Examiner	Masters	—	—	0	—	yes	—	1 yr.	5	3	4	8/20/70
				Psychologist	Doctorate	1	2	2	yes	no	no	2 yrs.				
Colorado	(L)	1961	1969	Psychological Assistant	Masters	2	2	2	—	yes	no	1 yr.	7	2	3	7/1/63
				Psychologist	Doctorate											
Connecticut	(L)	1945	1969	Psychologist	Doctorate	—	—	1	yes	yes	no	1 yr.	3	2	5	6/24/69
Delaware	(L)	1962		Practice of Psychology	Doctorate	2	2	2	yes	yes	yes	2 yrs.	6	1	3	6/11/64
District of Columbia	(L)	1971		Practice of Psychology	Doctorate	2	—	2	yes	yes	no	2 yrs.	5	0	3	4/8/72
Florida	(C)	1961	1981	Psychological Services	Doctorate	1	2	2	yes	yes	yes	2 yrs.	5	2	4	12/31/81
Georgia	(L)	1951		Practice of Applied Psychology	Doctorate	—	—	1	yes	yes	yes	2 yrs.	5	1	5	5/1/53
Hawaii	(L)	1967		Practice of Psychology	Doctorate	—	1	1	—	yes	no	2 yrs.	5	2	2	6/6/68
Idaho	(L)	1963		Practice of Psychology	Doctorate	—	—	2	—	yes	no	1 yr.	3	0	3	7/1/64
Illinois	(C)	1963		Psychologist	Doctorate	1	2	2	—	yes	no	2 yrs.	5	0	5	8/15/71
Indiana	(C)	1969	1981	Psychologist in Private Practice	Doctorate	1	—	2	yes	yes	no	2 yrs.	5	1	3	7/1/72
Iowa	(L)	1974	1981	Clinical Psychologist	Doctorate	1	1	2	yes	yes	no	1 yr.	5	1	3	7/1/83
				Practice of Psychology	Doctorate	1	1	1	—	yes	no	1 yr.				1976
Kansas	(L)	1967		Psychologist	Doctorate	1	2	2	—	no	yes	2 yrs.	2	1	3	7/1/69
Kentucky	(L)	1948		Practice of Psychology	Doctorate	1	—	1	yes	yes	no	3 yrs.	4	1	4	7/1/65
				Certificand	Masters							3 yrs.				
Louisiana	(L)	1964		Psychologist	Doctorate	1	2	2	yes	yes	yes	1 yr.	5	0	3	7/1/66

Maine	(L)	1953		Psychologist	Doctorate	–	–	2	–	yes	no	2 yrs.	5	1	5	10/1/68
				Psychologist Examiner	Masters	–	1	1	–	yes	no	2 yrs.				
Maryland	(L)	1957	1981	Psychologist	Doctorate	1	1	2	yes	yes	yes	1 yr.	5	1	3	12/31/59
Massachusetts	(L)		1971	Psychologist	Doctorate	1	1	2	yes	yes	no	2 yrs.	5	0	5	12/31/73
Michigan	(L)	1959	1978	Psychologist	Doctorate	–	–	2	–	yes	yes	1 yr.	5	3	4	
				(Limited License)	Doctorate/ Masters	–	–	–								10/1/80
Minnesota	(L)	1951	1973	Consulting Psychologist	Doctorate	2	2	2	yes	yes	no	2 yrs.	7	4	4	7/1/75
				Psychologist	Masters	2	–	2	yes	yes	no	2 yrs.				
Mississippi	(L)	1966		Psychologist	Doctorate	1	1	1	yes	yes	no	1 yr.	5	0	3	7/1/67
Missouri	(L)	1977		Psychologist	Doctorate	–	–	–	–	yes	no	1 yr.	5	0	5	4/28/78
					Masters	–	–	3	–	yes	no	1 yr.				
Montana	(L)	1971		Practice of Psychology	Doctorate	1	–	2	yes	yes	no	1 yr.	3	1	3	1/1/73
Nebraska	(L)	1967	1978	Practice of Psychology	Doctorate	–	–	0	–	yes	no	1 yr.	5	0	5	1/1/71
				(also specialty certification for clinical)												1/1/79
Nevada	(L)	1963		Practice of Psychology	Doctorate	1	4	1	–	yes	yes	2 yrs.	4	1	3	7/1/64
New Hampshire	(L)	1957	1981	Psychologist	Doctorate	1	2	2	yes	yes	no	1 yr.	5	2	3	7/1/82
				Associate Psychologist, Psychological Assistant	Masters	5	5	5	–	yes	no	1 yr.				7/1/82
New Jersey	(L)	1966		Practice of Professional Psychological Services	Doctorate	1	2	2	yes	yes	no	2 yrs.	7	3	3	1/1/68
New Mexico	(C)	1963		Psychologist	Doctorate	2	2	2	yes	yes	yes	1 yr.	5	1	3	12/31/64
New York	(C)	1956		Psychologist	Doctorate	–	2	2	yes	yes	no	2 yrs.	12	1	5	7/1/59
North Carolina	(L)	1967		Practicing Psychologist	Doctorate	2	2	2	yes	yes	no	1 yr.	5	0	3	7/1/69
				Psychological Associate	Masters	–	–	0	–	yes		1 yr.				
North Dakota	(L)	1967		Psychologist	Doctorate	–	–	0	yes	yes	no	1 yr.	5	0	3	7/1/68
Ohio	(L)	1972		Practice of Psychology	Doctorate	1	2	2	yes	yes	no	2 yrs.	6	1	5	11/22/76
	(L)	1972	1972	Practice of School Psychology	Masters	3	1	4	–	yes	no	2 yrs.				
Oklahoma	(L)	1965		Practice of Psychology	Doctorate	2	2	2	yes	yes	no	1 yr.	5	0	3	6/28/66
Oregon	(L)	1973		Practice of Psychology	Doctorate	–	2	2	yes	yes	yes	1 yr.	7	2	3	1/1/74
	(L)	(Limited)		Psychologist Associate	Masters	–	3	–	–	yes						
Pennsylvania	(L)	1972		Practice of Psychology	Doctorate	2	1	2	yes	yes	no	2 yrs.	7	2	3	5/23/72
					Masters	4	2	4	–	yes	no	2 yrs.				
Rhode Island	(C)	1969		Consulting Psychologist	Doctorate	1	2	2	yes	yes	no	1 yr.	4	1	3	12/31/70
South Carolina	(L)	1968		Practice of Psychology	Doctorate	1	2	2	yes	yes	no	2 yrs.	7	0	5	3/21/69
South Dakota	(L)	1976	1981	Practice of Psychology	Doctorate	2	–	2	–	yes	yes	2 yrs.	4	1	3	1/1/82

CHART 1 *(concluded)*
A summary of laws regulating the practice of psychology through (L) Licensure or (C) Certification

State		First approved in	Major amendments	Coverage	Requirements								Examining board			
					Educational requirements	Post degree	Supervision	Total experience	ABPP recognized	Mandatory examination	Continuing education for renewal	Renewal every	Psychology members	Public members	Terms	"Grandparenting" ends
Tennessee	(L)	1953		Psychologist	Doctorate	–	–	1	yes	yes	no	perm.	5	0	5	7/1/55
				Psychological Examiner	Masters			0								
Texas	(L)	1969	1975	Psychologist (also specialty certification for Health Service Provider)	Doctorate	1	1	2	yes	yes	yes	1 yr.	6	2	6	12/31/70
	(C)	1975	1981	Psychological Associate	Masters											
Utah	(L)	1959		Practice as Psychologist	Doctorate	1	2	2	no	yes	yes	1 yr.	5	0	5	12/31/62
Vermont	(L)	1976		Practicing Psychologist	Doctorate	2	2	3	yes	yes	yes	2 yrs.	3	2	5	6/30/77
				Psychological Associate	Masters	3	3	4	–	yes	yes	2 yrs.				
Virginia	(L)	1946	1966	Psychologist	Doctorate	2	2	2	yes	yes	yes	2 yrs.	5	0	5	none
			1966	Clincial Psychologist	Doctorate	2	2	2	yes	yes	yes	2 yrs.				
			1976	School Psychologist	Masters	4	2	4	yes	yes	no	2 yrs.				
Washington	(L)	1955		Practice of Psychology (also certification of qualification—limited licensure below doctorate)	Doctorate	1	1	1	yes	yes	yes	1 yr.	5	0	3	6/10/66
				Psychological Assistant												
West Virginia	(L)	1970		Practice of Psychology	Doctorate	1	1	1	yes	yes	yes	2 yrs.	5	1	3	11/12/70
					Masters	5	5	5	–	yes	yes	2 yrs.				
Wisconsin	(L)	1969	1979	Practice of Psychology	Doctorate	1	1	1	yes	no	no	2 yrs.	4	1	3	7/1/70
				School Psychologist	Masters											
Wyoming	(L)	1965		Practice of Psychology	Doctorate	–	–	0	yes	yes	yes	1 yr.	5	0	3	12/31/65
Canada																
Alberta	(C)	1960		Psychologist	Masters	–	–	0	–	no	no	–	8	0	1	4/11/62
British Columbia	(C)	1977		Psychologist	Doctorate	1	1	1	–	no	no	1 yr.	5	2	2	7/6/80

(450 clock hrs.)

Jurisdiction		Year	Title	Degree							Experience				Date
Manitoba	(C)	1966	Psychologist	Doctorate	2	2	2	—	—	—	1 yr.	7	0	2	12/31/72
New Brunswick	(L)	1980	Psychologist	Doctorate	1	1	1	—	yes	no	2 yrs.	5	0	2	6/1/71
Nova Scotia	(C)	1980	Psychologist	Masters	4	4	4	yes	yes	no	2 yrs.	5	0	3	12/18/84
				Doctorate	1	2	2	yes	yes	no	1 yr.				
Ontario	(C)	1960	Psychologist	Masters	4	4	4	—	yes	no	1 yr.	5	0	5	6/11/66
				Doctorate	1	1	1	—	—	no					
Quebec	(C)	1962	Psychologue	Doctorate	—	—	0	—	—	no	1 yr.	2	4	2	
				Masters	—	—	0	—	—	no					
Saskatchewan	(C)	1962	Registered Psychologist	Doctorate	—	—	0	yes	yes	—	1 yr.	5	0	2	12/31/66

Source: American Psychological Association, 1200 Seventeenth Street N.W., Washington, D.C. 20036. Reprinted by permission.

gist." Licensure laws do the same, but they also enumerate activities which constitute the practice of psychology for which a license is required, without regard to the title by which the practitioner is identified. State laws regulating psychological practice generally extend exemptions to members of other recognized professional groups employing psychological skills or techniques in their work, provided that they not identify themselves as "psychologists." Most psychology licensure and certification laws are generic in that they confer the same license for general practice upon psychologists whatever their field of applied specialization may be. The APA *Ethical Principles of Psychologists,* which are referenced by many state laws, serve to limit a psychologist's practice to their particular area of competence.

State examining boards

State laws regulating psychological practice are generally administered by a Board of Psychologist Examiners, which may include one or more "public" (nonpsychologist) members. Chart 1 serves to briefly summarize some of the key features of psychological practice legislation. For further information on admission to the licensure or certification process, contact the appropriate State Board. A list of State Board of Examiners is available through the APA Office of Professional Affairs.

Educational requirements

Most state laws establish that doctorate training in psychology or in a field of study ". . . . primarily psychological in nature" is the minimum requirement for the use of the title (noun) "psychologist" in the context of independent and unsupervised practice. Statutory recognition for training below the doctorate level is afforded in some states by use of the adjective "psychological" along with the term "assistant" or "associate." Ordinarily, psychological assistants or associates function under the supervision of a psychologist licensed or certified for independent and unsupervised practice.

Generally, degree programs held to be "primarily psychological" by State Boards of Examiners are earned in programs within institutions which are themselves accredited, or psychology programs within institutions wherein the institution has been accredited by one of the regional states institutional accrediting agencies. The APA currently accredits doctoral level programs in the recognized principal fields of applied psychology; namely, clinical, counseling, and school psychology.

Preliminary work which could lead to the implementation of a program to test a procedure for designating which programs train providers of psychological services goes forward at the time of this writing. The criteria under consideration for inclusion in the designation project are generally similar to those employed by the Council of National Register of Health Service Providers in determining *Register* listings. It is not intended that only "designated" programs imply entitlement to apply for a license or certificate to practice; graduates of other than designated programs would have the opportunity as they do now to present information to the State Boards of Examiners demonstrating the "primarily psychological" content of their training experience. Developoments relating to the "designation" project will be reported on in the APA *Monitor* as they occur. Students applying for graduate school and contemplating eventual licensure or certification will want to keep informed on the project.

For further information on individual psychology training programs (some of which lead to licensure/certification eligibility and others which do not), consult the APA *Graduate Study in Psychology.*

Scope of regulation

Laws regulating psychological practice ordinarily affect individuals identifying themselves to the public in the context of "fee-for-service" practice. Research and academic activities are also ordinarily exempt from regulation. Federal Civil Service and state civil service job classsifications often do not require state licensure or certification, although this may change in the years ahead. At their higher levels involving independent practitioner skills, the Federal Civil Service standards parallel state requirements for practice.

In some states separate licensure or certification programs have been established under state law for other professional specialties; for example, "marriage counseling" or "psychotherapist" certification. Just as psychology laws extend exemptions to other recognized groups, so too are psychologists licensed or certified for independent general practice exempted from these other regulatory programs.

State Departments of Education often certify school psychologists, trained to the masters level, for service within educational settings in most cases. Department of Education Certification as a School Psychologist does not constitute a license or certificate for the independent general practice of psychology.

Continuing education

State Examining Boards may require continuing education credits as one of the conditions of licensure or certificate renewal. The requirements are either in the licensing/certification law itself or are part of the administrative regulations developed by the board. At the time of this writing, several states not listed on Chart 1 are moving to implement continuing education requirements. In an additional number of states, amendments to the licensure/certification statute establishing continuing education requirements are contemplated. Check with your state board to determine the continuing education situation in your state.

The APA has established a continuing education sponsor approval program. While the program does not endorse or rate specific continuing education offerings, it does identify which continuing education sponsors meet APA standards in program design and development. Information on the sponsor approval program, and information relating to coutinuing education in general, is available through the APA Continuing Education Office.

Examination of candidates

Most State Boards of Examiners currently employ the standardized *Examination for Professional Practice in Psychology* in the course of administering licensure and certification programs. EPPP is developed by the Examination Committee of AASPB. State Boards may supplement the EPPP examination with written questions of their own or an oral examination. The EPPP is given each Spring and Fall. Applications for admission to the test should be made through the appropriate State Board of Examiners. While the APA does not review or approve examination preparatory courses, many workshops or home study courses are advertised in the *Monitor,* the official newspaper of the American Psychological Association. Pass/fail scores for the EPPP are set by the individual State Boards, as the admission requirements for licensure and certification vary somewhat from state to state.

American Board of Professional Psychology (ABPP) diplomate

Holders of the ABPP Diplomate automatically qualify for admission to the licensure or certification process in many states. The diplomate is conferred upon individuals who have successfully completed examination in one of the four principal fields of specialization in applied psychology: clinical, counseling, industrial/organizational, and school. Candidates for the ABPP diplomate must be trained to the doctoral level and have upwards of five years of experience, four of which shall be postdoctoral. For further information on the ABPP examination, contact: American Board of Professional Psychology, c/o Joseph Sanders, Ph.D., 2025 "I" Street, N.W., Suite 405, Washington, D.C. 20006 (202 833-2730).

National Register of Health Service Providers in Psychology

Since 1975 the National Register of Health Service Providers in Psychology has served to identify which generically licensed or certified psychologists are qualified in the area of health services. Current requirements for voluntary listing in the *Register* are: (1) doctoral degree in psychology; (2) two years of experience in a health setting; and (3) training in a psychology program meeting criteria approved by the *Register* Council. For further information on the National Register, contact: Council for the National Register of Health Service Providers in Psychology, 1200 17th Street, N.W., Washington, D.C. 20036.

Reciprocity

Formal reciprocal licensing or certification agreements between states have generally been discontinued. Most State Boards reserve the right to review credentials on a case-by-case basis. Should it be apparent that an individual was licensed or certified in another state with requirements reasonably similar to the new state of residence or practice, the application process may sometimes be foreshortened. Such a decision may be made only by the State Board administering the licensure or certification program.

Employment opportunities

A comprehensive listing of current employment opportunities in all fields of psychology (some specifying licensure/certification, others not) is provided in each month's issue of the American Psychological Association's official newspaper, the *Monitor.* The classified section is mailed separately just prior to the Convention double issue.

The APA provides an employment locator service to registrants at its annual meetings. Information on registration for the APA annual meetings appears in the Association's anchor journal, the *American Psychologist,* and in the *Monitor.*

Chart explanations

In addition to formal training, experience requirements have been established in most states. Of the total requirement, that portion which must be either "post degree" or earned under the supervision of a qualified psychologist is indicated. "ABPP Recognized" refers to the American Board of Professional Psychology diplomate. "Grandparenting" refers to the last date by which psychologists meeting previous standards for practice can apply for a license or certificate without submitting themselves to the credential review and examination process. "Grandparenting" generally occurs only at the time that a law regulating psychological practice has just been put into effect.

APPENDIX III

Intake forms for medicine, dentistry, and psychotherapy

A. Intake form for medicine*

PATIENT'S PERSONAL HISTORY FORM

NOTE: This is a confidential record and will be kept in this facility of your doctor's office. Information contained here will not be released to anyone without our authorization to do so

NAME _____ Age _____ Date _____

Occupation _____ Birth Place _____ Birth Date _____

Dr. _____ Date of last Physical Examination ___ _____
List all States and Countries _____
in which you have lived _____

Chief Complaints: (Please list all symptoms.)

1. _____ 3. _____
2. _____ 4. _____

Please answer each of the following questions by placing an (✓) in the "yes" box if your answer to the question is yes. or by placing an (✓) in the "no" box if your answer to the question is.no. Fill in "who" and "when" information when necessary.

FAMILY HISTORY

Has Any Blood Relative Ever Had:

Cancer, Including Leukemia	☐ NO	☐ YES	WHO _____
Tuberculosis	☐ NO	☐ YES	WHO _____
Diabetes	☐ NO	☐ YES	WHO _____
Heart Trouble	☐ NO	☐ YES	WHO _____
Heart Attack	☐ NO	☐ YES	WHO _____
High Blood Pressure	☐ NO	☐ YES	WHO _____
Stroke	☐ NO	☐ YES	WHO _____
Epilepsy	☐ NO	☐ YES	WHO _____
Bleeding Disorder	☐ NO	☐ YES	WHO _____
Asthma	☐ NO	☐ YES	WHO _____
Allergies	☐ NO	☐ YES	WHO _____
Liver Disease	☐ NO	☐ YES	WHO _____
Migraine Headaches	☐ NO	☐ YES	WHO _____
Alcoholism	☐ NO	☐ YES	WHO _____
Emphysema	☐ NO	☐ YES	WHO _____
Stomach or Duodenal Ulcer	☐ NO	☐ YES	WHO _____
Kidney Disease	☐ NO	☐ YES	WHO _____
Glaucoma	☐ NO	☐ YES	WHO _____
Sickle Cell Anemia	☐ NO	☐ YES	WHO _____

Family History (continued)

Other Anemia	☐ NO	☐ YES	WHO _____
Mental Illness	☐ NO	☐ YES	WHO _____
Suicide	☐ NO	☐ YES	WHO _____
Birth Defects	☐ NO	☐ YES	WHO _____
Other Serious Disease	☐ NO	☐ YES	WHO _____

PERSONAL HISTORY

Do You Smoke?   ☐ NO   ☐ YES
If Yes, What _____
How Much _____

Do You Drink?
Beer   ☐ NO   ☐ YES
Wine   ☐ NO   ☐ YES
Other Alcoholic
Beverages   ☐ NO   ☐ YES
How Much of Each? _____

Are You on a Special Diet?   ☐ NO   ☐ YES
What Diet? _____

	Living	Dead	Age at Death	Cause of Death
Father				
Mother				
Brother or Sister				
Husband or Wife				
Son or Daughter				

Form 1106 Briggs Corporation, Des Moines, Iowa 50306   Printed in U.S.A.

*Form reprinted with permission from the Briggs Corporation, Des Moines, Iowa 50306. For examples of other medical forms, the reader is invited to write to the Briggs Printing Division, 7887 University Boulevard, Des Moines, Iowa 50311.

DIAGNOSED DIFFICULTIES (continued)

Abnormal Chest X-Ray	☐ NO	☐ YES HAVE NOW	☐ YES PAST	WHEN _____
Heart Murmur as an Adult	☐ NO	☐ YES HAVE NOW	☐ YES PAST	WHEN _____
Abnormal Electrocardiogram	☐ NO	☐ YES HAVE NOW	☐ YES PAST	WHEN _____
Enlarged Heart	☐ NO	☐ YES HAVE NOW	☐ YES PAST	WHEN _____
Heart Attack	☐ NO	☐ YES HAVE NOW	☐ YES PAST	WHEN _____
Rheumatic Fever	☐ NO	☐ YES HAVE NOW	☐ YES PAST	WHEN _____
Angina	☐ NO	☐ YES HAVE NOW	☐ YES PAST	WHEN _____
High Blood Pressure	☐ NO	☐ YES HAVE NOW	☐ YES PAST	WHEN _____
Gall Stones	☐ NO	☐ YES HAVE NOW	☐ YES PAST	WHEN _____
Hepatitis	☐ NO	☐ YES HAVE NOW	☐ YES PAST	WHEN _____
Cirrhosis of Liver	☐ NO	☐ YES HAVE NOW	☐ YES PAST	WHEN _____
Stomach or Duodenal Ulcer	☐ NO	☐ YES HAVE NOW	☐ YES PAST	WHEN _____
Abnormal Stomach X-Ray	☐ NO	☐ YES HAVE NOW	☐ YES PAST	WHEN _____
Colon or Bowel Trouble	☐ NO	☐ YES HAVE NOW	☐ YES PAST	WHEN _____
Rectal Trouble	☐ NO	☐ YES HAVE NOW	☐ YES PAST	WHEN _____
Hemorrhoids or Piles	☐ NO	☐ YES HAVE NOW	☐ YES PAST	WHEN _____
Dysentery or Serious Diarrhea	☐ NO	☐ YES HAVE NOW	☐ YES PAST	WHEN _____
Kidney or Bladder Infection	☐ NO	☐ YES HAVE NOW	☐ YES PAST	WHEN _____
Kidney Stones	☐ NO	☐ YES HAVE NOW	☐ YES PAST	WHEN _____
Other Kidney Disease What? _____	☐ NO	☐ YES HAVE NOW	☐ YES PAST	WHEN _____
Anemia What Kind? _____	☐ NO	☐ YES HAVE NOW	☐ YES PAST	WHEN _____
Poor Blood Clotting	☐ NO	☐ YES HAVE NOW	☐ YES PAST	WHEN _____
Diabetes	☐ NO	☐ YES HAVE NOW	☐ YES PAST	WHEN _____
On Insulin How Much? _____	☐ NO	☐ YES		
Gout	☐ NO	☐ YES HAVE NOW	☐ YES PAST	WHEN _____
Overactive Thyroid	☐ NO	☐ YES HAVE NOW	☐ YES PAST	WHEN _____
Underactive Thyroid	☐ NO	☐ YES HAVE NOW	☐ YES PAST	WHEN _____
Goiter	☐ NO	☐ YES HAVE NOW	☐ YES PAST	WHEN _____
Broken Bones	☐ NO	☐ YES HAVE NOW	☐ YES PAST	WHEN _____
Varicose Veins	☐ NO	☐ YES HAVE NOW	☐ YES PAST	WHEN _____
Arthritis	☐ NO	☐ YES HAVE NOW	☐ YES PAST	WHEN _____
Polio	☐ NO	☐ YES HAVE NOW	☐ YES PAST	WHEN _____
Phlebitis	☐ NO	☐ YES HAVE NOW	☐ YES PAST	WHEN _____
Syphilis or V.D.	☐ NO	☐ YES HAVE NOW	☐ YES PAST	WHEN _____
Gonorrhea	☐ NO	☐ YES HAVE NOW	☐ YES PAST	WHEN _____
Recurrent Boils	☐ NO	☐ YES HAVE NOW	☐ YES PAST	WHEN _____
Other Skin Disease What Kind? _____	☐ NO	☐ YES HAVE NOW	☐ YES PAST	WHEN _____
Serious Depression	☐ NO	☐ YES HAVE NOW	☐ YES PAST	WHEN _____
Serious Emotional Problem	☐ NO	☐ YES HAVE NOW	☐ YES PAST	WHEN _____
Nervous Breakdown	☐ NO	☐ YES HAVE NOW	☐ YES PAST	WHEN _____

Women

Menstrual Difficulties	☐ NO	☐ YES HAVE NOW	☐ YES PAST	WHEN _____
Ovarian Cyst	☐ NO	☐ YES HAVE NOW	☐ YES PAST	WHEN _____
Other Gyn Problems What Kind? _____	☐ NO	☐ YES HAVE NOW	☐ YES PAST	WHEN _____
Age Periods Started _____				
Still Menstruating	☐ NO	☐ YES		
Age Periods Stopped _____				
Why Periods Stopped _____				
Are Your Periods Regular?	☐ NO	☐ YES _____		
Cystitis	☐ NO	☐ YES HAVE NOW	☐ YES PAST	WHEN _____
Mastitis	☐ NO	☐ YES HAVE NOW	☐ YES PAST	WHEN _____
Breast Cancer	☐ NO	☐ YES HAVE NOW	☐ YES PAST	WHEN _____
Other Breast Disease	☐ NO	☐ YES HAVE NOW	☐ YES PAST	WHEN _____
Number of Times Pregnant _____				
Number of Children _____				
Number of Miscarriages _____				

Men

Prostate Trouble	☐ NO	☐ YES HAVE NOW	☐ YES PAST	WHEN _____
Other Illness What? _____	☐ NO	☐ YES HAVE NOW	☐ YES PAST	WHEN _____

Personal History (continued)

Have You Lost Weight in the Past Year? ☐ NO ☐ YES

Do You Have Difficulty Sleeping? ☐ NO ☐ YES

Are You Overweight? ☐ NO ☐ YES

X-RAYS

Have You Had Any of these X-Rays? If Yes, When?

Chest	☐ NO	☐ YES	WHEN _____
Stomach	☐ NO	☐ YES	WHEN _____
Colon	☐ NO	☐ YES	WHEN _____
Gall Bladder	☐ NO	☐ YES	WHEN _____
Back	☐ NO	☐ YES	WHEN _____
Kidney	☐ NO	☐ YES	WHEN _____
Extremities	☐ NO	☐ YES	WHEN _____
Other	☐ NO	☐ YES	WHEN _____

Have You Ever Had X-Ray Treatments? ☐ NO ☐ YES WHEN _____

IMMUNIZATIONS

Have You Been Immunized Against:

Small Pox	☐ NO	☐ YES	LAST SHOT _____
Tetanus	☐ NO	☐ YES	LAST SHOT _____
Polio (shots or oral vaccine)	☐ NO	☐ YES	LAST SHOT _____
Measles	☐ NO	☐ YES	LAST SHOT _____
German Measles	☐ NO	☐ YES	LAST SHOT _____
Other _____	☐ NO	☐ YES	LAST SHOT _____

ALLERGIES

Are You Allergic to Any of the Following?

Penicillin	☐ NO	☐ YES
Sulfa	☐ NO	☐ YES
Other Antibiotics	☐ NO	☐ YES
Any Other Drug or Medicine	☐ NO	☐ YES
Any Food	☐ NO	☐ YES
Nail Polish or Cosmetic	☐ NO	☐ YES
Other _____	☐ NO	☐ YES

MEDICINES

Are You Taking Any Medicines Regularly Now? _____ ☐ NO ☐ YES WHAT _____

Medicines (continued)

Have You Ever Taken:

Insulin	☐ NO	☐ YES	WHEN _____
Cortisone	☐ NO	☐ YES	WHEN _____
Thyroid Medicine	☐ NO	☐ YES	WHEN _____
Male or Female Hormones	☐ NO	☐ YES	WHEN _____
Blood Pressure Medicine	☐ NO	☐ YES	WHEN _____
Tranquilizers or Sedatives	☐ NO	☐ YES	WHEN _____
Birth Control Pills	☐ NO	☐ YES	WHEN _____
Other	☐ NO	☐ YES	WHEN _____

DEVICES

Do You Use:

Eyeglasses	☐ NO	☐ YES
Contact Lenses	☐ NO	☐ YES
Hearing Aid	☐ NO	☐ YES
Dentures	☐ NO	☐ YES
Neck Brace	☐ NO	☐ YES
Back Brace	☐ NO	☐ YES
Other Brace	☐ NO	☐ YES
Artificial Limb	☐ NO	☐ YES
Truss	☐ NO	☐ YES
Pacemaker	☐ NO	☐ YES
I.U.D.	☐ NO	☐ YES
Diaphragm	☐ NO	☐ YES
Other Device	☐ NO	☐ YES

OPERATIONS

Have You Had Any of these Operated Upon:

Tonsils	☐ NO	☐ YES	WHEN _____
Appendix	☐ NO	☐ YES	WHEN _____
Gall Bladder	☐ NO	☐ YES	WHEN _____
Stomach	☐ NO	☐ YES	WHEN _____
Small Intestine	☐ NO	☐ YES	WHEN _____
Kidney	☐ NO	☐ YES	WHEN _____
Colon	☐ NO	☐ YES	WHEN _____
Thyroid	☐ NO	☐ YES	WHEN _____
Hernia (Rupture)	☐ NO	☐ YES	WHEN _____

Women

Breast	☐ NO	☐ YES	WHEN _____
Uterus	☐ NO	☐ YES	WHEN _____
Ovaries	☐ NO	☐ YES	WHEN _____

Men

Prostate	☐ NO	☐ YES	WHEN _____
Other	☐ NO	☐ YES	WHEN _____

DIAGNOSED DIFFICULTIES

Do You Now, or Have You in the Past, Had Any of the Following:

Migraine Headaches	☐ NO	☐ YES HAVE NOW	☐ YES PAST	WHEN _____
Epilepsy or Convulsions	☐ NO	☐ YES HAVE NOW	☐ YES PAST	WHEN _____
Stroke	☐ NO	☐ YES HAVE NOW	☐ YES PAST	WHEN _____
Glaucoma	☐ NO	☐ YES HAVE NOW	☐ YES PAST	WHEN _____
Cataracts	☐ NO	☐ YES HAVE NOW	☐ YES PAST	WHEN _____
Blindness Either Eye	☐ NO	☐ YES HAVE NOW	☐ YES PAST	WHEN _____
Ear Infections	☐ NO	☐ YES HAVE NOW	☐ YES PAST	WHEN _____
Deafness	☐ NO	☐ YES HAVE NOW	☐ YES PAST	WHEN _____
Asthma	☐ NO	☐ YES HAVE NOW	☐ YES PAST	WHEN _____
Hay Fever	☐ NO	☐ YES HAVE NOW	☐ YES PAST	WHEN _____
Chronic Bronchitis	☐ NO	☐ YES HAVE NOW	☐ YES PAST	WHEN _____
Emphysema	☐ NO	☐ YES HAVE NOW	☐ YES PAST	WHEN _____
Tuberculosis	☐ NO	☐ YES HAVE NOW	☐ YES PAST	WHEN _____

SYSTEM REVIEW
Do You Have Any of the Following Complaints:

General

Fever	☐ NO	☐ YES
Chills	☐ NO	☐ YES
Aches or Pains	☐ NO	☐ YES
General Weakness	☐ NO	☐ YES
Memory Loss	☐ NO	☐ YES
Swollen Glands	☐ NO	☐ YES
Easy Bruising	☐ NO	☐ YES

Head

Blurred Vision Not Corrected by Glasses	☐ NO	☐ YES
Double Vision	☐ NO	☐ YES
Light Flashes	☐ NO	☐ YES
Halos Around Lights	☐ NO	☐ YES
Pain in Your Eyes	☐ NO	☐ YES
Ear Pain	☐ NO	☐ YES
Drainage from Ear	☐ NO	☐ YES
Hearing Difficulty or Deafness	☐ NO	☐ YES
Buzzing or Ringing in Ears	☐ NO	☐ YES
Nosebleeds Not Due to Injuries	☐ NO	☐ YES
Sinus Trouble	☐ NO	☐ YES
Difficulty Swallowing	☐ NO	☐ YES
Mouth, Tooth or Tongue Problem	☐ NO	☐ YES
Persistent Hoarseness	☐ NO	☐ YES
Severe Headaches	☐ NO	☐ YES
Other_____	☐ NO	☐ YES

Skin

Changing Mole	☐ NO	☐ YES
Rash	☐ NO	☐ YES
Yellow Skin	☐ NO	☐ YES
Other Skin Problem _____	☐ NO	☐ YES

Neck

Swelling	☐ NO	☐ YES
Lumps	☐ NO	☐ YES
Stiffness	☐ NO	☐ YES
Other _____	☐ NO	☐ YES

Chest, Heart, Lungs

Shortness of Breath	☐ NO	☐ YES
Poor Exercise Tolerance	☐ NO	☐ YES
Fluttering of Heart	☐ NO	☐ YES
Unusual Heartbeat	☐ NO	☐ YES
Chest Pain or Pressure Attacks	☐ NO	☐ YES
Frequent Cough	☐ NO	☐ YES
Coughing Up Blood	☐ NO	☐ YES
Wheezing	☐ NO	☐ YES
Night Sweats	☐ NO	☐ YES
Swollen Ankles	☐ NO	☐ YES
Leg Cramps	☐ NO	☐ YES
Other _____	☐ NO	☐ YES

Gastrointestinal

Poor Appetite	☐ NO	☐ YES
Indigestion or Heartburn	☐ NO	☐ YES
Difficulty Swallowing	☐ NO	☐ YES
Nausea or Vomiting	☐ NO	☐ YES
Vomiting Blood	☐ NO	☐ YES
Abdominal Pain or Cramps	☐ NO	☐ YES
Abdominal Swelling	☐ NO	☐ YES
Diarrhea	☐ NO	☐ YES
Constipation	☐ NO	☐ YES
Change in Bowel Habits	☐ NO	☐ YES
Pass Blood from Rectum	☐ NO	☐ YES
Black, Tar-like Bowel Movements	☐ NO	☐ YES
Other_____	☐ NO	☐ YES

Kidney

Blood in Urine	☐ NO	☐ YES
Pain or Burning While Urinating	☐ NO	☐ YES
Difficulty Passing Urine	☐ NO	☐ YES
Difficulty Controlling Urine	☐ NO	☐ YES
Getting Up at Night to Urinate	☐ NO	☐ YES
Other_____	☐ NO	☐ YES

Genitalia

Women

Breast Lump	☐ NO	☐ YES
Discharge from Nipple	☐ NO	☐ YES
Other Breast Problem	☐ NO	☐ YES
Vaginal Discharge	☐ NO	☐ YES
Vaginal Bleeding or Spotting (not with periods)	☐ NO	☐ YES
Hot Flashes	☐ NO	☐ YES
Pain with Intercourse	☐ NO	☐ YES
Possibly Pregnant	☐ NO	☐ YES
Change in Periods	☐ NO	☐ YES
Pain Not Associated with Periods	☐ NO	☐ YES
Other _____	☐ NO	☐ YES

Men

Breast Lump	☐ NO	☐ YES
Discharge from Penis	☐ NO	☐ YES
Sore on Penis	☐ NO	☐ YES
Lump in Testicles	☐ NO	☐ YES
Difficulty Having Erections	☐ NO	☐ YES
Other _____	☐ NO	☐ YES

Neuromuscular

Weakness in Arm or Leg	☐ NO	☐ YES
Difficulty with Balance	☐ NO	☐ YES
Dizzy Spells	☐ NO	☐ YES
Fainting Spells	☐ NO	☐ YES
Speech Difficulty	☐ NO	☐ YES
Other _____	☐ NO	☐ YES

Bones—Joints

Painful Joints	☐ NO	☐ YES
Swollen Joints	☐ NO	☐ YES
Loss of Muscle Strength	☐ NO	☐ YES
Lump or Swelling in Muscle	☐ NO	☐ YES
Lump on Bone	☐ NO	☐ YES
Back Pain	☐ NO	☐ YES
Other _____	☐ NO	☐ YES

Endocrine

Thirsty All the Time	☐ NO	☐ YES
Cold Most of the Time	☐ NO	☐ YES
Too Warm Most of the Time	☐ NO	☐ YES
Unusually Tired or Sluggish	☐ NO	☐ YES
Unusually Jumpy or Nervous	☐ NO	☐ YES

Psychologic

Do You Find Your Life:

Generally Unsatisfactory	☐ NO	☐ YES
Too Demanding	☐ NO	☐ YES
Boring	☐ NO	☐ YES
Satisfactory	☐ NO	☐ YES

Do You Worry About:

Money	☐ NO	☐ YES
Job	☐ NO	☐ YES
Marriage	☐ NO	☐ YES
Home Life	☐ NO	☐ YES
Children	☐ NO	☐ YES

Do You:

Cry Easily	☐ NO	☐ YES
Feel Inferior to Others	☐ NO	☐ YES
Feel Shy	☐ NO	☐ YES
Feel Things Often Go Wrong	☐ NO	☐ YES
Often Feel Depressed	☐ NO	☐ YES
Have Irrational Fears	☐ NO	☐ YES
Feel Anxious or Upset	☐ NO	☐ YES

Have You:

Seriously Considered Suicide	☐ NO	☐ YES
Attempted Suicide	☐ NO	☐ YES

B. Intake form for pedodontia*

Health Record

CHILD'S NAME _____

NICKNAME _____ AGE _____ GRADE _____

SCHOOL _____

CHILD'S INTERESTS _____ HOBBIES _____

FATHER'S NAME _____ HOME PHONE _____

STREET ADDRESS _____ CITY _____ STATE _____ ZIP _____

FATHER EMPLOYED BY _____ PHONE _____

BUSINESS ADDRESS _____

PRESENT POSITION _____ HOW LONG HELD _____

MOTHER'S NAME _____ HOME PHONE _____

STREET ADDRESS _____ CITY _____ STATE _____ ZIP _____
(if different from father's)

MOTHER EMPLOYED BY _____ PHONE _____

BUSINESS ADDRESS _____

PRESENT POSITION _____ HOW LONG HELD _____

PURPOSE OF THIS APPOINTMENT _____

IN CASE OF EMERGENCY, WHOM SHOULD BE NOTIFIED _____ PHONE _____

WHO WILL PAY THIS ACCOUNT _____
(if other than parent)

PARENT'S SOCIAL SECURITY NUMBER _____

IF USING CHARGE CARD, NAME _____ CARD NO. _____

IF WELFARE, YOUR NUMBER _____ COUNTY OF _____

HAS THERE EVER BEEN ANY INJURY TO ANY OF YOUR CHILD'S TEETH BY FALL, BLOW, BUMP, OR OTHERWISE?

IF SO, DESCRIBE _____

HAS ANY MEMBER OF YOUR FAMILY HAD AN UNUSUAL DENTAL HISTORY SUCH AS MISSING OR EXTRA TEETH?

YES _____ NO _____

WHAT DO YOU THINK OF THE CONDITION OF YOUR CHILD'S MOUTH? _____

_____

OTHER CHILDREN IN FAMILY _____
    (Names and ages)

WHOM MAY WE THANK FOR REFERRING YOUR CHILD _____

COMMENTS: _____

_____

_____

*Form designed by Burton A. Jordan, D.D.S. and reprinted with his permission.

DATE OF BIRTH_____ DATE OF LAST HEALTH CARE EXAMINATION _____

FOR WHAT_____

HAS CHILD BEEN HOSPITALIZED IN LAST 5 YEARS _____ IF SO, FOR WHAT_____

_____

HAS CHILD EVER HAD:

	YES NO		YES NO
ANEMIA	— —	RHEUMATIC FEVER	— —
DIABETES	— —	HEART MURMUR	— —
EPILEPSY	— —	CHICKEN POX	— —
HEPATITIS	— —	MUMPS	— —
ALLERGIES TO:	— —	MEASLES	— —
PENICILLIN	— —	ABNORMAL HEART CONDITION	— —
LOCAL ANESTHETIC	— —	ABNORMAL BLOOD PRESSURE	— —
MEDICATION OR DRUGS	— —	ABNORMAL BLEEDING FROM A CUT	— —

IF ALLERGIES TO MEDICATIONS OR DRUGS, INDICATE WHICH ONES _____

IS CHILD TAKING ANY MEDICATION_____IF SO, FOR WHAT _____

OTHER PHYSICAL CONDITIONS_____

_____

_____

_____

IS CHILD RECEIVING OTHER HEALTH CARE NOW_____IF SO, NATURE OF CARE _____

NAME OF PHYSICIAN_____ PHONE NO._____

ADDRESS_____

MAY WE REQUEST YOUR CHILD'S HEALTH RECORDS IF NECESSARY _____ YES _____ NO _____

TO WHOM SHOULD WE ADDRESS REQUEST_____

_____

THIS INFORMATION WAS GIVEN BY_____ DATE _____

DO YOU WISH US TO PERFORM ROUTINE TREATMENT IN YOUR ABSENCE?   YES _____ NO _____

DO YOU WISH US TO PERFORM EMERGENCY TREATMENT IN YOUR ABSENCE? YES _____ NO _____

C. Intake form for adult psychotherapy

CONFIDENTIAL
PATIENT INFORMATION

Patient name (print) _____ Date first seen _____

Address _____ Date of birth _____

_____ zip _____ Home phone (_____) _____

Occupation _____ Business phone (_____) _____

Address _____ zip _____

Please check:
( ) single   ( ) married   ( ) remarried   ( ) separated   ( ) divorced   ( ) widow(er)

Education (highest grade completed): _____

Spouse's name _____ Date of birth _____

Address and phone if different from above _____

_____

Occupation _____ Business phone (_____) _____

Address _____ zip _____

Family: names, ages, birthdates, grade if in school

_____

_____

_____

_____

Health Insurance Company _____ ID# _____

Other health insurance _____ ID# _____

Name of family physician (address and phone) _____

_____

Current medications of patient _____

Allergies of patient _____

Name of doctor or facility providing previous mental health services:

_____

Patient referred by: _____

Comments: _____

PLEASE NOTE OFFICE CANCELLATION POLICY:
   Each appointment time is reserved for only one person or family. Reserved time must be cancelled at least 24 hours ahead to avoid full charge.

D. Intake form for child psychotherapy

CONFIDENTIAL
CHILD PATIENT INFORMATION

Patient name (print) _____ Date first seen _____

Address _____ Date of birth _____

_____ zip _____ Home phone (_____) _____

School name, grade, name of teacher _____

_____

Family: Siblings names, ages, birthdates, grade if in school

_____

_____

_____

_____

Parent or guardian _____ Date of birth _____

Address and phone (if different from above) _____

_____

Occupation _____ Business phone (_____) _____

Address _____ zip _____

Please check:
( ) single   ( ) married   ( ) remarried   ( ) separated   ( ) divorced   ( ) widow(er)

Spouse's name _____ Date of birth _____

Address and phone (if different from above) _____

_____

Occupation _____ Business phone (_____) _____

Address _____ zip _____

Health Insurance Company _____ ID# _____

Other health insurance _____ ID# _____

Name of patient's physician (or family physician), address and phone:

_____

Current medications of patient _____

Allergies of patient _____

Name of doctor or facility providing previous mental health services:

_____

Patient referred by: _____

Comments: _____

PLEASE NOTE OFFICE CANCELLATION POLICY:
    Each appointment time is reserved for only one person or family. Reserved time must be cancelled at least 24 hours ahead to avoid full charge.

E. Newborn data base form*

NEWBORN DATA BASE

Prenatal History

Grav _____ Para _____ AB _____
_____

General health during pregnancy
_____

Problems _____
_____
_____

Prenatal care started _____
Drugs: Vits _____ Iron _____
Other _____
Attitude toward pregnancy:
Mother _____
Father _____

Labor and Delivery

Duration _____
Type _____
Complications _____

Neonatal History

Gestation _____ Apgar _____
WT _____/_____% HT _____/_____%
OFC _____/_____%
Nursery course _____
_____
_____

First feeding at _____
Responses to infant _____
_____
_____
_____

Feeding _____
_____

Family Planning

Attended prenatal classes _____
Attended postpartum classes _____
Plans for birth control _____
_____

Family History

Mother's marital status _____
Age: Mother _____ Father _____
Siblings:

Age	Sex	Health

Diseases

Maternal	Paternal

Social History

Infant's primary caretaker _____
Mother's work plans _____
_____
Supportive resources _____
_____
_____

Father currently _____
Remarks _____
_____
_____
_____

Teaching

Growth and development _____
Nutrition _____
Safety _____
Infant care _____
Illness _____

History obtained _____ (date) by _____ (signature)
Name _____ Sex _____ Place of birth _____
SS # _____ Birthdate _____

*For use by nurse practitioners. Form designed by Linda Levett, R.N. and reprinted with her permission.

APPENDIX IV

Examples of
third-party payer forms

A. Office management form for third–party payment

Monthly insurance submissions

Date submit	Company	Patient	Dates of service	ID # and/or SS #	Profile	Deduc-tible	Amount due	Amount paid	Date paid

B. Standard inquiry form for third–party payers

STANDARD INQUIRY FORM

To: _____

_____ Fiscal Intermediary

_____ Name and Address

_____

Re: Patient/Beneficiary Name: _____

Sponsor Social Security No. or VA File No. _____

Sponsor Name: _____

Street Address: _____

City/State/Zip Code: _____

Area and Telephone No.: _____

Date(s) of Service: _____

Provider Name/Address: _____

_____

Control Number (If already processed attach copy of CEOB):

_____

Statement of Problem:

From: _____

_____ Inquirer Name,

_____ Address and Telephone

_____ Number

C. Universal third–party payment form

FORM APPROVED
OMB NO 86 R0012

HEALTH INSURANCE CLAIM FORM
Read Instructions Before Completing or Signing This Form

☐ MEDICARE   ☐ MEDICAID   ☐ CHAMPUS   ☐ OTHER

PATIENT & INSURED (*SUBSCRIBER*) INFORMATION

1 Patient's Name (First Name Middle Initial Last Name)	2 Patient's Date of Birth Month Day Year	3 Insured's Name (First Name Middle Initial Last Name)
4 Patient's Address (Street City State Zip Code)	5 Patient's Sex Male ☐ Female ☐	6 Insured's Medicare or Champus ID Number
	7 Patient's Relationship To Insured Self Spouse Child Other	8 Insured's Group No (Or Group Name)
Telephone Number		
9 Other Health Insurance Coverage Enter **MEDICAL ASSISTANCE CASE NUMBER** or Name of Policy Holder Plan Name Number and Address	10 Was Condition Related To A Patient's Employment Yes / No B Auto Accident Yes / No C Other Accident Yes / No	11 Insured's Address (Street City State Zip Code) Active Duty Station (Champus Only) Telephone Number
12 PATIENT'S OR AUTHORIZED PERSON'S SIGNATURE (Read back before signing) I Authorize the Release of any Medical Information Necessary to Process the Claim and Request Payment of Medicare Medicaid or Champus Benefits Either to Myself or to the Party Who Accepts Assignment Below Signed _____ Date _____		13 I Authorize Payment of Medical Benefits to Undersigned Physician or Supplier for Service Described Below Signed (Insured or Authorized Person)

PHYSICIAN OR SUPPLIER INFORMATION

14 Date of Illness (First Symptom) or Injury (Accident) or Pregnancy (LMP)	15 Date First Consulted You for this Condition	16 Has Patient Ever Had Same or Similar Symptoms? Yes / No	16a If an Emergency Check Here
17 Date Patient Able to Return to Work	18 Dates of Total Disability From _____ Through _____	18a Dates of Partial Disability From _____ Through _____	
19 Name of Referring Physician or Other Source (e g Public Health Agency) ☐ Private Practice or ☐ Military Service		20 For Services Related to Hospitalization Give Hospitalization Dates Admitted _____ Discharged _____	
21 Name & Address of Facility Where Services Rendered (If Other Than Home or Office)		22 Was Laboratory Work Performed Outside your Office? Yes ☐ No ☐ Charges _____	
23 Diagnosis or Nature of Illness or Injury Relate Diagnosis to Procedure in Column D by Reference Numbers 1 2 3 etc or DX Code A 1 2 3		23B EPSDT Yes / No Family Planning Yes / No Abortion Yes / No Sterilization Yes / No Prior Authorization No _____	

24 A Date of Service From — To	B Place of Service	C TOS	D Fully Describe Procedures Medical Services or Supplies Furnished for Each Date Given Procedure Code (Identify) (Explain Unusual Services or Circumstances)	E Diagnosis Code	F Charges	G Days/ Times/ Units	H Amount Paid By Other Insurance

25 Signature of Physician or Supplier (I Certify that the Statements on the Reverse Apply to this Bill and Are Made a Part Hereof) Signed _____ Date _____	26 Accept Assignment (Government Claims Only) (See Back) Yes ☐ No ☐	27 Total Charge	28 Amount Paid	29 Balance Due
	30 Your Social Security No	31 Physician's or Supplier's Name, Address, Zip Code & Telephone No		
32 Your Patient Account No	33 Your Employer ID No			
		Provider No		
Place of Service and Type of Service (TOS) Codes on Back Remarks		Approved by AMA Council on Medical Service Approved by The Health Care Financing Administration & Champus HCFA 1500/CHAMPUS 501 (2)		

Form provided through courtesy of CHAMPUS division of Blue Cross/Blue Shield of Rhode Island.

APPENDIX V

Preoperative disclosure form

Carl E. Alberto, D.D.S., Ltd.

Diplomate
American Board
of
Oral & Maxillofacial Surgery

324 Greenview Lane
Dorsett, Rhode Island 20888
937-0505

GENERAL INFORMATION CONCERNING COMPLICATIONS

The following general complications were reviewed in detail by Dr. Carl E. Alberto concerning my total treatment plan on

NO TREATMENT

1. Future or continued jaw joint problems such as pain, limitation of opening, arthritis, degenerative joint disease, clicking, popping, joint noise, and general problems with chewing and speech.
2. Continued or future periodontal disease manifested by gingivitis, periodontitis, loss of bony support to the teeth, loss of teeth, and a higher instance of tooth decay.
3. The present malocclusion without treatment can become worse with time thereby contributing to those problems listed in 1 and 2.
4. If the remaining upper and lower teeth are lost, the use of complete or partial dentures may be difficult in terms of chewing and speech.
5. Emotional considerations as they relate to the patient's self-image.

COMPLICATIONS AS A RESULT OF TREATMENT:

1. Damage to teeth secondary to the orthodontics or surgery resulting in root canals, capping of the teeth, or loss of the teeth.
2. Dental relapse as a result of orthodontic tooth movement.
3. Skeletal relapse due to technical problems with surgery, bone healing, pre-existing periodontal disease, infection, and growth considerations.
4. Damage to the nerves supplying sensation to the upper lip, side of the nose, upper cheek, lower eyelid, upper teeth and surrounding soft tissues, lower teeth and surrounding soft tissues, lower lip, soft tissue chin. This can result in total lack of normal feeling or that of slight tingling sensation.
5. Hemorrhage during surgery requiring more complicated surgery, blood transfusions, and possible secondary hepatitis or latent bleeding necessitating a return to surgery for adequate control.
6. Infection can result in severe swelling, lack of bone healing, or major complications such as a brain abscess.
7. Swelling may be mild to severe and will last for a minimum of 10 days. Bruising may occur resulting in discoloration of the skin of the face and the mucosa of the oral cavity for three to four weeks.
8. Pain may be mild to severe necessitating prolongation of the hospital stay and the use of narcotics to control the symptoms.

9. *Major* complications of anesthesia such as allergic reactions, high fevers, heart standstill requiring appropriate resuscitative procedures and possible death.
10. *Major* surgical complications such as hemorrhage or infection with obstruction of the airway which could result in death.
11. Other surgical complications which can alter the healing process resulting in relapse manifested by a return of the malocclusion or a return of the facial asymmetry.
12. Immediate postoperative surgical complications necessitating a return to surgery prior to discharge.
13. Postoperative treatment functional and esthetic problems necessitating another surgical procedure.
14. Orthodontics, favorable or unfavorable growth, and surgical considerations may result in an alteration in our final surgical treatment plan either increasing or decreasing the amount of required surgery.
15. Other complications or problems which may arise during treatment not discussed at this time.
16. All quoted fees are estimates and they are subject to change prior to surgery.

I understand that while the Doctor will attempt to achieve the desired results for me there is no insurance, warranty, or guarantee, explicit or implied of specific results or cure associated with my treatment. I also realize that the management of my problem is multifaceted-multifactorial and one cannot always predict the patient's response to treatment. It was explained to me that the Doctor will strive to achieve the optimum result but the ideal result cannot always be realized.

Signature of patient: *Carl E. Alberto, D.D.S.*

_____   _____

Signature of guardian: *Witness:*

_____   _____

                                                  Date:

                                                  _____

This form was developed by Albert E. Carlotti, Jr., D.D.S. and is reprinted with his permission.

APPENDIX VI

Release of information form

```
┌─────────────────────────────────────────────────────────────┐
│                   RELEASE OF INFORMATION                      │
│                                                               │
│   I  hereby  authorize  _____ to  release  to │
│   _____ any and/or all medical, psychological, or educa- │
│   tional information pertaining to _____.       │
│                                                               │
│   Signature _____ Date _____            │
│   Witness  _____ Date _____             │
│                                                               │
└─────────────────────────────────────────────────────────────┘
```

APPENDIX VII

Annotated list of associations for allied health professionals*

ACADEMY OF PSYCHOLOGISTS IN MARITAL SEX AND FAMILY THERAPY (APMSFT)

246 Virginia Ave.   Phone: (201) 886-1090
Ft. Lee, NJ 07024   Anthony J. Vilhotti, Exec. Dir.
Founded: 1958. Members: 431. Local Groups: 4. Psychologists holding membership in the American Psychological Association (see separate entry) who are interested in family, marital, and sex therapy. To teach, conduct research, and practice in the field of marital sex and family therapy. Compiles statistics. Bestows awards. Maintains speakers bureau and conducts specialized education programs. Committees: Ethics; Publications; Research; Standards. Publications: (1) Newsletter, quarterly; (2) The Relationship, 4–5/year; (3) Directory, biennial. Formerly: (1975) Academy of Psychologists in Marital Counseling; (1980) Academy of Psychologists in Marital and Family Therapy. Convention/Meeting: annual—in conjunction with American Psychological Association.

AMERICAN ASSOCIATION OF NURSE ANESTHETISTS (AANA)

216 W. Higgins Rd.   Phone: (312) 692-7050
Park Ridge, IL 60068   Nancy A. Fevold, Exec. Dir.
Founded: 1931. Members: 22,000. Staff: 25. State Groups: 52. Active registered nurses who have taken an approved 24-month course in anesthesiology and passed a qualifying examination. To advance the art and science of anesthesiology and to develop educational standards and techniques. Sponsors continuing education. Presents annual Agatha Hodgins Award for outstanding accomplishment. Councils: Accreditation; Certification; Practice; Recertification. Publications: (1) News Bulletin, monthly; (2) Journal, bimonthly. Formerly: (1939) National Association of Nurse Anesthetists. Convention/Meeting: annual—always August or September. 1984 Chicago, IL; 1985 Aug. 17–22, Anaheim, CA.

AMERICAN ACADEMY OF OCCUPATIONAL MEDICINE (AAOM)

150 N. Wacker Dr.   Phone: (312) 782-2166
Chicago, IL 60606   Donald L. Hoops, Ph.D., Exec. Dir.
Founded: 1946. Members: 740. Physicians whose primary interest is in some phase of occupational medicine. Promotes maintenance and improvement of the health of industrial workers. Publications: (1) Journal of Occupational Medicine, monthly; (2) Membership Directory, annual. Convention/Meeting: annual—usually fall.

AMERICAN ACADEMY OF PEDODONTICS (AAP)

211 E. Chicago Ave., Suite 1036   Phone: (312) 337-2169
Chicago, IL 60611   Merle C. Hunter, Exec. Dir.
Founded: 1947. Members: 2,400. Professional society of dentists whose practice is limited to children; teachers and researchers in pedodontics. Sponsors graduate student pedodontic award program. Publications: (1) Newsletter, bimonthly; (2) Pediatric Dentistry (journal), quarterly. Convention/Meeting: annual—always May. 1984 May 26-29,

---

*The list of organizations is reprinted by permission of the Gale Research Company, Detroit, and is derived from Denise Akey, ed., *Encyclopedia of Associations,* vol. 1, 17th ed. (copyright © 1959, 1961, 1964, 1968, 1970, 1972, 1973, 1975, 1976, 1977, 1978, 1979, 1980, 1981, and 1982). By Gale Research Company. The organizations listed were selected where membership exceeded 1,000 and/or annotations indicated broad applicability to allied health professionals. The reader is invited to explore the original publication which contains an exhaustive listing as well as listings for specific geographic areas.

Scottsdale, AZ; 1985 May 25-28, Washington, DC; 1986 May 24-27, Colorado Springs, CO.

AMERICAN ACADEMY OF PERIODONTOLOGY (AAP)

211 E. Chicago Ave.   Phone: (312) 787-5518
Chicago, IL 60611   Marilyn C. Holmquist, Exec. Sec.
Founded: 1914. Members: 4,100. Staff: 8. Professional society of dentists specializing in treatment of supporting and surrounding tissues of the teeth and their diseases. Committees: Dental; Foreign Relations; Periodontal Pathology Center; Public and Professional Relations; Research in Periodontology; Student Loan. Publications: (1) Journal of Periodontology, monthly; (2) Newsletter, bimonthly; (3) Roster of Members, annual. Absorbed: (1967) American Society of Periodontists. Convention/Meeting: annual—usually October. 1984 Sept. 19-22, New Orleans, LA; 1985 Sept. 11-14, San Francisco, CA; 1986 Oct. 22-25, Cleveland, OH.

AMERICAN ACADEMY OF PSYCHOANALYSIS (AAP)

30 E. 40th St.   Phone: (212) 679-4105
New York, NY 10016   Vivian Mendelsohn, Adm. Dir.
Members: 897. Staff: 3. Psychoanalysts (740) are fellows of the Academy; associates (99) are scientists or educators; candidates (58). Seeks to develop communication among psychoanalysts and persons in other disciplines in science and the humanities; provides a forum for inquiry into the phenomena of individual motivation and social behavior; encourages and supports research.

AMERICAN ASSOCIATION FOR MARRIAGE AND FAMILY THERAPY (AAMFT)

924 W. Ninth   Phone: (714) 981-0888
Upland, CA 91786   Dr. C. Ray Fowler, Exec. Dir.
Founded: 1942. Members: 9,000. Staff: 10. Regional Groups: 45. Professional society of marriage and family therapists. Assumes a major role in maintaining and extending the highest standards of excellence in this field. Has 13 accredited training centers throughout the U.S. and provides a nationwide marriage and family therapy referral service from its national office. Individuals serve as international affiliates in 13 foreign countries. Publications: (1) Newspaper, bimonthly; (2) Journal, quarterly; (3) Membership Register, biennial. Formerly: (1970) American Association of Marriage Counselors; (1978) American Association of Marriage and Family Counselors. Convention/Meeting: annual—1984 Oct. 10-13, New York City.

AMERICAN BOARD OF PROFESSIONAL PSYCHOLOGY (ABPP)

2025 I St., N.W., Suite 405   Phone: (202) 833-2730
Washington, DC 20006   Joseph R. Sanders, Ph.D., Exec. Dir.
Founded: 1947. Trustees: 10. Staff: 3. Certification board which conducts oral examinations and awards diplomas to advanced specialist in four professional specialties: Clinical Psychology, Industrial and Organizational Psychology, Counseling Psychology, and School Psychology. Candidates must have five years of qualifying experience in psychological practice. Presents Distinguished Professional Achievement Award annually. Publications: (1) Manual for Oral Examinations, annual; (2) Policies and Procedures, annual; (3) Directory of Diplomates, triennial. Formerly: (1968) American Board of

Examiners in Professional Psychology. Convention/Meeting: annual—always August or September.

AMERICAN COLLEGE OF DENTISTS (ACD)

7315 Wisconsin Ave., Suite 352N   Phone: (301) 986-0555
Bethesda, MD 20814   Dr. Gordon H. Rovelstad, Exec. Dir.
Founded: 1920. Members: 4,800. Staff: 5. Local Groups: 37. Dentists and others serving in capacities related to the dental profession. Seeks to advance the standards of the profession of dentistry. Bestows W. J. Gies Award annually in recognition of exceptional service to the profession by a Fellow. Committees: Conduct; Education and Research. Publications: Journal of the ACD, quarterly. Convention/Meeting: annual—1984 Oct. 20, Atlanta, GA; 1985 Nov. 2, San Francisco, CA; 1986 Nov. 6, St. Louis, MO.

AMERICAN DENTAL ASSOCIATION (ADA)

211 E. Chicago Ave.   Phone: (312) 440-2500
Chicago, IL 60611   John M. Coady, Exec. Dir.
Founded: 1859. Members: 137,000. Staff: 435. State Groups: 54. Local Groups: 488. Professional society of dentists. To encourage the improvement of the health of the public and to promote the art and science of dentistry. Inspects and accredits dental schools and schools for dental hygienists, assistants and laboratory technicians. Conducts research programs at ADA Health Foundation Research Institute. Produces most of the dental health education material used in the United States. Sponsors National Children's Dental Health Month and science fair programs. Compiles statistics on personnel, practice, dental care needs and attitudes of patients related to dental health. Maintains library of 35,000 volumes; biographical records of U.S. dentists, past and present; collection of published and original documentary material of historical interest to the profession; library is in charge of developing uniform standards of nomenclature in the field of dental science. Maintains 16 councils including: Communications; Dental Research; and Insurance. Publications: (1) News, 40/year; (2) Dental Abstracts, monthly; (3) Journal, monthly; (4) Journal of Endodontics, monthly; (5) Special Care in Dentistry, bimonthly; (6) Index to Dental Literature, quarterly; (7) Directory, annual; (8) Accepted Dental Therapeutics, biennial; (9) Dentist's Desk Reference: Materials, Instruments and Equipment, triennial. Absorbed: (1897) Southern Dental Association. Formerly: (1922) National Dental Association. Convention/Meeting: annual—usually October or November. 1984 Oct. 20–23, Atlanta, GA; 1985 Nov. 2–5, San Francisco, CA; 1986 Oct. 18–21, Miami Beach, FL.

AMERICAN GROUP PSYCHOTHERAPY ASSOCIATION (AGPA)

1995 Broadway, 14th Fl.   Phone: (212) 787-2618
New York, NY 10023   Marsha Block, Exec. Officer
Founded: 1942. Members: 3,000. Staff: 6. Local Groups: 25. Psychiatrists, psychologists, social workers, psychiatric nurses and other mental health professionals who meet specific educational and professional requirements. Presents awards. Sponsors educational and research programs. Maintains 14 committees including: Children and Adolescents; Legislative Information and Social Issues; and Standards and Ethics. Publications: (1) International Journal of Group Psychotherapy, quarterly; (2) Newsletter, quarterly; (3) Membership Directory, biennial; also publishes Consumer's Guide to Group Psychotherapy, Brief History of the Association 1943–1968; Guidelines for Training of Group Psychotherapists; and membership directory. Convention/Meeting: annual—always February. 1984 location undecided; 1985 New York City.

AMERICAN MEDICAL ASSOCIATION (AMA)

535 N. Dearborn St.   Phone: (312) 751-6000
Chicago, IL 60610   James H. Sammons, M.D., Exec. V. Pres.
Founded: 1847. Members: 282,000. Staff: 894. State and Territorial Groups: 56.
County Medical Societies: 1,950. Physicians who are members in good standing in 56
state and territorial associations. Disseminates scientific information to members and the
public. Informs members on significant medical and health legislation on state and national levels and represents profession with Congress and governmental agencies. Cooperates in setting standards for medical schools, hospitals, residency programs, and continuing medical education courses. Offers physician placement service and counseling
on practice management problems. Operates library which lends material and provides
specific medical information to physicians. Maintains councils which make policy studies and recommendations on all levels of medical education, scientific affairs, medical
practice, legislation, judicial, by-laws and long-range planning. Ad-hoc committees are
formed for such topics as health care planning, principles of medical ethics, and others.
Publications: (1) American Medical News, weekly; (2) Journal of the AMA, weekly; (3)
American Journal of Disease of Children, monthly; (4) Archives of Dermatology,
monthly; (5) Archives of General Psychiatry, monthly; (6) Archives of Internal Medicine, monthly; (7) Archives of Opthalmology, monthly; (8) Archives of Otolaryngology,
monthly; (9) Archives of Neurology, monthly; (10) Archives of Pathology and Laboratory Medicine, monthly; (11) Archives of Surgery, monthly. Convention/Meeting: semiannual—1984 June 17–21, Chicago, IL; 1985 June 16–20, Chicago, IL.

AMERICAN MEDICAL ASSOCIATION AUXILIARY (AMAA)

535 N. Dearborn St.   Phone: (312) 751-6166
Chicago, IL 60610   Hazel Lewis, Exec. Dir.
Founded: 1922. Members: 82,000. Physicians' spouses. Purpose is to assist physicians
in protecting and improving public health and in providing quality medical care. Sponsors Project Bank, an information clearinghouse of community projects initiated by auxiliaries across the country, including programs on child abuse, VD awareness and services to the aging. Promotes health education and health careers for students through its
Career Day programs and health fairs. Contributes to the AMA Education and Research
Foundation (see separate entry). Sponsors Shape Up for Life Campaign which is aimed
at keeping Americans healthy by making them aware that proper diet, exercise and
stress management are vital to good health and fitness. Committees: American Medical
Association Education and Research Foundation; Health Projects; Legislation. Publications: (1) Direct Line Newsletter, bimonthly; (2) Facets, 5/year. Formerly: (1975)
Woman's Auxiliary to the American Medical Association. Convention/Meeting: annual—
always Chicago, IL. 1984 June 17–20.

AMERICAN NURSES' ASSOCIATION (ANA)

2420 Pershing Rd.   Phone: (816) 474-5720
Kansas City, MO 64108   Myrtle K. Aydelotte, Ph.D., Exec. Dir.
Founded: 1896. Members: 165,000. Staff: 140. State Groups: 53. Local Groups: 860.
Professional organization of registered nurses. Sponsors American Nurses' Foundation
(research in nursing) and American Academy of Nursing (see separate entries); sponsors
Nurses Coalition for Action in Politics, which endorses candidates who support nursing
interests and encourages political involvement among nurses. Presents Pearl McIlver
Public Health Award for outstanding contribution to public health nursing; Mary Maho-

ney Award for significant contribution toward opening opportunities in nursing to minority groups; Jessie M. Scott Award for excellence in nursing practice, education and research; Shirley Titus Award for outstanding contribution to economic and general welfare program; and honorary nursing practice, recognition and membership awards. Maintains hall of fame. Commissions: Economic and General Welfare; Human Rights; Nursing Education; Nursing Research; Nursing Services. Committees: Ethics. Councils: Advisory; Continuing Education; High Risk Perinatal Nurses; Intercultural Nursing; Nurse Researchers; Nursing Administration; Nursing Home Nurses; Primary Health Care Nurse Practitioners; Specialists in Psychiatric and Mental Health Nursing. Divisions: Community Health; Gerontological; Maternal and Child Health; Medical-Surgical; Psychiatric and Mental Health Nursing. Publications: (1) American Journal of Nursing, monthly; (2) The American Nurse, monthly; (3) Facts About Nursing, annual; (4) Biennial Reports to House of Delegates; (5) Proceedings of the the House of Delegates, biennial; also publishes Nursing Standards and professional literature. Affiliated with: International Council of Nurses. Formerly: (1911) Nurses Associated Alumnae of United States and Canada. Convention/Meeting: biennial—always June.

AMERICAN ORTHOPSYCHIATRIC ASSOCIATION (ORTHO)

1775 Broadway
New York, NY 10019
Phone: (212) 586-5690
Marion F. Langer, Ph.D. Exec. Dir.
Founded: 1924. Members: 8,000. Staff: 16. Psychiatrists, psychologists, psychiatric social workers, and members drawn from related fields of anthropology, sociology, education, nursing and allied professions. To unite and provide a common meeting ground for those engaged in the study and treatment of problems of human behavior. To foster research and spread information concerning scientific work in the field of human behavior, including all forms of abnormal behavior. Maintains Public Issues Council. Study Groups: Aging; Children's Rights and Parent's Rights; Confidentiality of Health and Social Service Records; Cultural Pluralism; Mental Health in Schools; Native Americans. Publications: American Journal of Orthopsychiatry, quarterly; also publishes newsletter, membership directory and monographs.

AMERICAN PSYCHIATRIC ASSOCIATION (APA)

1700 18th St., N.W.
Washington, DC 20009
Phone: (202) 797-4900
Melvin Sabshin, M.D., Med. Dir.
Founded: 1844. Members: 26,000. Staff: 140. Regional Groups: 75. Psychiatrists united to further the study of the nature, treatment and prevention of mental disorders. Assists states in formulating programs to meet mental health needs; develops standards for psychiatric facilities; compiles and disseminates facts and figures about psychiatry; furthers psychiatric education and research; maintains library. Commissions: Psychiatric Therapies. Councils: Aging; Children, Adolescents and Their Families; International Affairs; Law and Psychiatric Practice; Medical Education and Career Development; Mental Health Services; National Affairs; Research and Development. Publications: (1) Psychiatric News, semimonthly; (2) American Journal of Psychiatry, monthly; (3) Hospital and Community Psychiatry, monthly; (4) Membership Directory, triennial; also publishes books and pamphlets. Formerly: (1892) Association of Medical Superintendents of American Institutions for Insane; (1921) American Medico-Psychological Association. Convention/Meeting: annual—always May. 1984 Los Angeles, CA; 1985 Dallas, TX.

AMERICAN PERSONNEL AND GUIDANCE ASSOCIATION (APGA)

Two Skyline Pl., Suite 400
5203 Leesburg Pike   Phone: (703) 820-4700
Falls Church, VA 22041   Charles L. Lewis, Exec. V. Pres.

Founded: 1952. Members: 39,000. Staff: 50. State Groups: 53. Professional society of guidance and personnel workers in elementary and secondary schools, higher education, community agencies and organizations, government, industry, and business. Maintains special library of 5,000 books and pamphlets. Maintains placement service for members. Committees: Commission on Human Rights; Ethical Practices; Federal Relations; Insurance Trust; International Education; Placement Service Review; Professional Preparation and Standards; Research Awards. Divisions: American College Personnel Association; American Mental Health Counselors Association (see separate entry); American Rehabilitation Counseling Association; American School Counselor Association; Association for Counselor Education and Supervision; Association for Humanistic Education and Development; Association for Measurement and Evaluation in Guidance; Association for Non-White Concerns in Personnel and Guidance; Association for Religious and Value Issues in Counseling (see separate entry); Association for Specialists in Group Work; National Employment Counselors Association; National Vocational Guidance Association; Public Offender Counselor Association. Publications: (1) Guidepost (newsletter), 18/year; (2) Personnel and Guidance Journal, 10/year; (3) Journal of College Student Personnel, bimonthly; (4) School Counselor, 5/year; (5) Counseling and Values, quarterly; (6) Counselor Education and Supervision, quarterly; (7) Humanist Educator, quarterly; (8) Journal of ANWC, quarterly; (9) Journal of Employment Counseling, quarterly; (10) measurement and Evaluation in Guidance, quarterly; (11) Rehabilitation Counseling Bulletin, 5/year; (12) Vocational Guidance, quarterly; (13) AMHCA Journal, semiannual; also publishes Public Offender Counselor Association Journal of Offending Counseling. Convention/Meeting: annual—1984 Houston, TX; 1985 New York City; 1986 Los Angeles, CA.

AMERICAN PSYCHOANALYTIC ASSOCIATION (APsaA)

One E. 57th St.   Phone: (212) 752-0450
New York, NY 10022   Helen Fischer, Adm. Dir.

Founded: 1911. Members: 2,667. Local Groups: 36. Professional association of medically oriented psychoanalysts who have graduated or are currently attending an accredited institute. To establish and maintain standards for the training of psychoanalysts and for the practice of psychoanalysis; to foster the integration of psychoanalysis with other branches of medicine; and to encourage research. Publications: (1) Journal, quarterly; (2) Newsletter, quarterly; (3) Roster, annual; also publishes Glossary of Psychoanalytic Terms and Concepts and material on psychoanalytic education and research. Convention/Meeting: semiannual—always May and December. 1984 May 2-6, San Diego, CA and Dec. 19-23 New York City; 1985 May 15-19, San Antonio, TX or Denver, CO and Dec. 18-22, New York City.

AMERICAN PSYCHOLOGICAL ASSOCIATION (APA)

1200 17th St., N.W.   Phone: (202) 833-7600
Washington, DC 20036   Michael Pallak, Ph.D., Exec. Officer

Founded: 1892. Members: 50,000. Staff: 200. State Groups: 53. Scientific and professional society of psychologists and educators; students participate as Student in Psychology subscribers. To advance psychology as a science, a profession, and as a means of promoting human welfare. Boards: Convention Affairs; Education and Training; Policy and Planning; Professional Affairs; Publications and Communications; Scientific Affairs; Social and Ethical Responsibility. Divisions: Adult Development and Aging; Child and Youth Services; Clinical Psychology; Community Psychology; Consulting Psychology; Consumer Psychology; Counseling Psychology; Developmental Psychology; Educational Psychology; Evaluation and Measurement; Experimental Analysis of Behavior; Experimental Psychology; General Psychology; Health Psychology; History of Psychology; Humanistic Psychology; Hypnosis; Industrial and Organizational Psychology; Mental Retardation; Military Psychology; Neuropsychology; Personality and Social Psychology; Philosphical Psychology; Physiological and Comparative Psychology; Population Psychology; Psychoanalysis; Psychologists Interested in Religious Issues; Psychologists in Public Service; Psychology and the Arts; Psychology of Women; Psychopharmacology; Psychotherapy; Rehabilitation Psychology; School Psychology; Society of Engineering Psychologists (see separate entry); Society for the Psychological Study of Social Issues (see separate entry); State Psychological Association Affairs; Teaching of Psychology. Publications: (1) American Psychologist, monthly; (2) Contemporary Psychology, monthly; (3) Employment Bulletin, monthly; (4) Journal of Personality and Social Psychology, monthly; (5) Monitor (newspaper), monthly; (6) Psychological Abstracts, monthly; (7) Developmental Psychology, bimonthly; (8) Journal of Abnormal Psychology, bimonthly; (9) Journal of Applied Psychology, bimonthly; (10) Journal of Comparative and Physiological Psychology, bimonthly; (11) Journal of Consulting and Clinical Psychology, bimonthly; (12) Journal of Counseling Psychology, bimonthly; (13) Journal of Educational Psychology, bimonthly; (14) Journal of Experimental Psychology: Learning, Memory, and Cognition, bimonthly; (15) Professional Psychology, bimonthly; (16) Psychological Bulletin, bimonthly; (17) Psychological Review, bimonthly; (18) Journal of Experimental Psychology; Animal Behavior Process, quarterly; (19) Journal of Experimental Psychology: General, quarterly; (20) Journal of Experimental Psychology: Human Perception and Performance, quarterly; (21) Journal Supplement Abstract Service, quarterly; also publishes Biographical Directory and Membership Register. Affiliated with: Psi Chi, the National Honorary Society in Psychology. Absorbed: Psychologists Interested in the Advancement of Psychotherapy; (1976) Psychologists Interested in Religious Issues. Convention/Meeting: annual—1984 Toronto, ON, Canada; 1985 Los Angeles, CA; 1986 Washington, DC.

AMERICAN SOCIETY FOR ADOLESCENT PSYCHIATRY (ASAP)

24 Green Valley Rd.   Phone: (215) 566-1054
Wallingford, PA 19086   Mary Staples, Exec. Sec.
Founded: 1967. Members: 1,700. Staff: 1. Local Groups: 20. Qualified psychiatrists who are interested in adolescents. Works to provide for the exchange of psychiatric knowledge, to encourage the development of adequate training facilities, and to stimulate research in the psychopathology and treatment of adolescents. Conducts workshops at annual scientific meetings. Consults with national organizations interested in the welfare of youth. Bestows awards; holds occasional symposia on topics relating to adolescent psychiatry. Publications: (1) Newsletter, quarterly; (2) Annals of Adolescent Psychiatry, annual; (3) Membership Directory, biennial. Convention/Meeting: annual—always May. 1984 April 29–May 1, New York City. Also holds biennial Pan-American Forum.

AMERICAN PSYCHOLOGY-LAW SOCIETY (AP-LS)

c/o Stephen O. Morse
Univ. of Southern California Law Center
University Park
Los Angeles, CA 90007   Stephen O. Morse, Pres.
Founded: 1968. Members: 550. Objectives are: to promote exchanges between the disciplines of psychology and law in regard to areas of mutual interest such as teaching, research, administration of justice, jurisprudence, and other matters at the psychology-law interface; to promote research relevant to legal problems using psychological knowledge and methods and to promote psychological research using the legal setting and related legal research techniques; to promote education of lawyers at all levels regarding psychology, and of psychologists at all levels regarding the law; to promote legislation and social policies consistent with current states of psychological knowledge; to promote the effective use of psychologists in the processes and setting of the law. Publications: (1) Journal of Law and Human Behavior, quarterly; (2) Newsletter, quarterly. Convention/Meeting: biennial conference.

AMERICAN SOCIETY OF CLINICAL HYPNOSIS (ASCH)

2250 E. Devon Ave., Suite 336   Phone: (312) 297-3317
Des Plaines, IL 60018   William F. Hoffman, Jr., Exec. Dir.
Founded: 1957. Members: 4,200. Staff: 6. State Groups: 15. Local Groups: 25. Physicians, dentists and psychologists with a doctoral degree. Brings together professional people in medical, dental and psychological fields using hypnosis; sets up standards of training; conducts teaching sessions and workshops at basic and advanced levels. Through its affiliate, ASCH-Education and Research Foundation (see separate entry), offers instruction on clinical hypnosis, various simple forms of psychotherapy and psychodynamics. Cooperates with all scientific disciplines in regard to use of hypnosis. Publications: (1) News Letter, 8/year; (2) American Journal of Clinical Hypnosis, quarterly; (3) Directory, annual. Convention/Meeting: annual scientific meeting—1984 Oct. 28–Nov. 3, Portland, OR; 1985 Oct. 14–19, New York, NY; 1986 San Diego, CA.

AMERICAN SOCIETY OF CLINICAL ONCOLOGY (ASCO)

435 N. Michigan Ave., Suite 1717   Phone: (312) 644-0828
Chicago, IL 60611   Alfred VanHorn, III, Exec. Dir.
Founded: 1964. Members: 3,300. Experienced physicians and paramedical personnel who have a predominant interest in the diagnosis and total care of patients with neoplastic diseases and who are directly involved in and responsible for the care of such patients. Presents the Karnovsky Memorial Lecture Awards. Publications: Directory, biennial. Convention/Meeting: annual—1984 May 6–8, Toronto, ON, Canada.

AMERICAN SOCIETY OF LAW AND MEDICINE (ASLM)

765 Commonwealth Ave., 16th Fl.   Phone: (617) 262-4990
Boston, MA 02215   A. Edward Doudera, Exec. Dir.
Founded: 1972. Members: 2,300. Staff: 10. Physicians, attorneys, health care management executives, nurses, insurance company personnel, members of the judiciary and all others interested in medicolegal relations and health law. Purpose is to continue medicolegal education through publications, conferences and information clearinghouse. Maintains speakers bureau, photocopy service and Sagall Library of Law, Medicine and

Health Care of over 2,000 volumes. Bestows annual Honorary Life Membership for distinguished achievements in the field of medicolegal education; sponsors annual student essay competition. Publications: (1) Nursing, Law and Ethics, 10/year; (2) Law, Medicine and Health Care, 6/year; (3) Medicolegal News, 6/year; (4) American Journal of Law and Medicine, quarterly; Formerly: (1973) Massachusetts Society of Law and Medicine.

ASSOCIATION FOR ADVANCEMENT OF BEHAVIOR THERAPY (AABT)

420 Lexington Ave.   Phone: (212) 682-0065
New York, NY 10170   Mary Jane Eimer, Exec. Dir.
Founded: 1966. Members: 3,300. Foreign and State Groups: 20. Psychiatrists and psychologists; about 5 percent of membership is made up of social workers, dentists, medical engineers, physiotherapists and other professionals interested in the issues, problems and development of the general field of behavior modification, with specific emphasis on the clinical applications. Sponsors training program and lectures for professionals and semi-professionals; maintains speaker's bureau; handles referrals for the public to locate behavior therapists in the area; and arranges for communication between behavior therapists interested in specific problems or information. Bestows annual Presidents New Research Award. AABT branches hold training meetings, workshops, seminars, case demonstrations and discussion groups. Committees: Continuing Education; Public Education; Publications. Publications: (1) The Behavior Therapist (mini journal), 5/year; (2) Behavior Therapy, 5/year; (3) Behaviorial Assessment Journal, quarterly; (4) Membership Directory, biennial; also publishes AVU Directory and Training Directory. Formerly: (1968) Association for Advancement of the Behavioral Therapies. Convention/Meeting: annual.

ASSOCIATION TO ADVANCE ETHICAL HYPNOSIS (AAEH)

60 Vose Ave.   Phone: (201) 762-3132
South Orange, NJ 07079   Maxwell M. Kaye, O.D., Pres.
Founded: 1955. Members: 1,500. Staff: 3. Practitioners of all the healing arts, educators, police officers, attorneys, lay technicians. To establish a code of ethics in the practice of hypnosis; to expose and discourage malpractice and the use and granting of non-academic titles and degrees; to oppose the restriction of hypnosis to members of special professional groups. Conducts three-phase examination (written, oral and practical) and certifies members as hypno-technicians. Bestows awards; maintains speakers bureau. Conducts research programs. Committees: Education; Ethics and Standards. Publications: Suggestion (newsletter), bimonthly. Convention/Meeting: annual.

ASSOCIATION FOR ADVANCEMENT OF PSYCHOLOGY (AAP)

1200 17th St., N.W., Suite 200   Phone: (202) 466-5757
Washington, DC 20036   Clarence J. Martin, Exec. Dir.
Founded: 1974. Members: 6,000. Staff: 7. Members of the American Psychological Association (see separate entry) or other national psychological associations, students of psychology, and organizations primarily psychological in nature. Purposes are to advance psychology and to represent the interests of all psychologists (professional, social and scientific) in the public policy arena. Publications: Advance (newsletter), monthly. Affiliated with: American Psychological Association. Absorbed: (1975) Council for the Advancement of Psychological Professions and Sciences. Convention/Meeting: annual.

ASSOCIATION OF EXISTENTIAL PSYCHOLOGY AND PSYCHIATRY (AEPP)

c/o Dr. Louis DeRosis
40 E. 89th St.
New York, NY 10028

Phone: (212) 348-3500
Dr. Louis DeRosis, Sec.

Founded: 1960. Members: 1,700. Staff: 3. Psychiatrists, psychologists, social workers, sociologists, theologians, teachers, college and university professors, philosophers, and others interested in a "multidimensional dialogue among all the disciplines which further the nontechnological aspects of human existence." Sponsors public lectures, a seminar, and study groups. Provides referral service for existential therapy. Publications: Review of Existential Psychology and Psychiatry, 3/year. Convention/Meeting: semiannual—always November and January.

ASSOCIATION OF HALFWAY HOUSE ALCOHOLISM PROGRAMS OF NORTH AMERICA (AHHAP)

786 E. Seventh St.
St. Paul, MN 55106

Phone: (612) 771-0933
William Ennis, Office Mgr.

Founded: 1966. Members: 1,000. Staff: 4. State Groups: 50. Halfway house corporations, staff, board members and individuals closely related to the halfway house movement. Charitable organization dedicated to educating and serving halfway house programs through technical assistance, consultant services, workshops, conferences, publications and similar services. Disseminates information and materials; compiles statistics and offers specialized education. Publications: (1) Communications and Services Newsletter, 10/year; (2) Counselors on Alcoholism Newsletter, 10/year; (3) Women's Task Force Newsletter, 8/year; (4) Conference Proceedings, annual; (5) Membership Directory, annual; also publishes statistical data. Convention/Meeting: annual conference.

AMERICAN ASSOCIATION OF MEDICAL ASSISTANTS (AAMA)

One E. Wacker Dr.
Chicago, IL 60601

Phone: (312) 944-2722
Ina L. Yenerich, Exec. Dir.

Founded: 1956. Members: 18,000. Staff: 16. State Groups: 47. Local Groups: 600. Assistants, receptionists, secretaries, bookkeepers, nurses and laboratory personnel employed in the offices of physicians and other medical facilities. Activities include a certification program consisting of study and an examination, passage of which entitles the individual to a certificate as a Certified Medical Assistant. Conducts accreditation of one and two-year programs in medical assisting in conjunction with the Committee on Allied Health Education and Accreditation and the American Medical Association (see separate entry). Provides assistance and information to institutions of higher learning desirous of initiating courses for medical assistants. Awards scholarships. Offers continuing education to assistants who cannot return to school and guided study courses in anatomy, terminology, physiology, human relations and specimen collection and preparation. Awards Continuing Education Units for selected educational programs. Maintains small library of textbooks and a reference list. Committees: International Relations; Legislation; Professional Advancement; Public Relations. Boards: Certification; Continuing Education; Curriculum Review. Publications: (1) The Professional Medical Assistant (journal), bimonthly; (2) Intercom (newsletter), irregular. Convention/Meeting: annual—always fall.

ASSOCIATION FOR HUMANIST SOCIOLOGY (AHS)

Dept. of Sociology
St. Lawrence University   Phone: (315) 379-6213
Canton, NY 13617   Stuart Hills, Sec.
Founded: 1976. Members: 500. Sociologists and other persons interested in humanistic sociology. Provides a forum for sociologists concerned with the value-related aspects of sociological theory, research and professional life. Seeks to extend the boundaries of humanist sociology by exploring connections between sociology and other disciplines. Committees: Editorial and Publications. Publications: (1) The Humanist Sociologist (newsletter), quarterly; (2) Humanity and Society, quarterly. Convention/Meeting: annual.

CENTER FOR MEDICAL CONSUMERS AND HEALTH CARE INFORMATION (CMCHCI)

237 Thompson St.   Phone: (212) 674-7105
New York, NY 10012   Arthur Levin, Dir.
Founded: 1976. Staff: 3. Purpose is to encourage people to make a critical evaluation of all information received from health professions; to use medical services more selectively and to understand the limitations of modern medicine; and to show people that lifestyle choices such as smoking, exercise habits and nutritional practices have more effect on health than access to medical care. Conducts research and publishes results; runs self-care workshops. Maintains medical library for laypeople containing over 1,000 volumes. Maintains telephone health library of over 140 tapes covering a variety of health topics which may be heard over the phone. Publications: Health Facts, monthly.

CONSUMER COALITION FOR HEALTH (CCH)

P.O. Box 50088   Phone: (202) 638-5828
Washington, DC 20004   Mark Kleiman, Exec. Dir.
Founded: 1977. Members: 600. Staff: 2. National and local consumer organizations, health planning agencies (100) and concerned individuals (500). Aims to create a climate where community health interests take precedence over special interests. Provides national advocacy in Congress, the agencies and the courts to promote consumer interests in health planning; gives assistance to consumers involved in public health policy decision making; provides public education programs to stimulate public interest in the health care delivery system. Publications: Consumer Health Action Network (newsletter), bimonthly.

NATIONAL ASSOCIATION OF SOCIAL WORKERS (NASW)

1425 H St., N.W., Suite 600   Phone: (202) 628-6800
Washington, DC 20005   Chauncey Alexander, Exec. Dir.
Founded: 1955. Members: 90,000. Staff: 125. State Groups: 55. Regular members are persons who hold a minimum of a baccalaureate degree in social work. Associate members are persons engaged in social work who have a baccalaureate degree in another field. Student members are persons enrolled in accredited (by the Council on Social Work Education) graduate or undergraduate social work programs. Purpose is to promote the quality and effectiveness of social work practice by: advancing sound social policies and programs and utilizing the professional knowledge and skills of social work

to "alleviate sources of deprivation, distress and strain"; setting professional standards; conducting study and research; improving professional education; publication and interpretation to the community. Maintains a library of 4,000 volumes. Presents National Public Citizen of the Year and National Social Worker of the Year awards. Administrative Units: Academy of Certified Social Workers; Publications Editorial Office. Publications: (1) Advocate for Human Services, monthly; (2) News, monthly (except August and December); (3) Social Work, bimonthly; (4) Health and Social Work, quarterly; (5) Practice Digest, quarterly; (6) Social Work in Education, quarterly; (7) Social Work Research and Abstracts, quarterly; also publishes Encyclopedia of Social Work, Directory of Professional Social Workers and various books and pamphlets. Formed by Merger of: American Association of Group Workers; American Association of Medical Social Workers; American Association of psychiatric Social Workers; American Association of Social Workers; Association for the Study of Community Organization; National Association of School Social Workers; Social Work Research Group. Convention/ Meeting: biennial delegate assembly and professional symposium.

NATIONAL LEAGUE FOR NURSING (NLN)

Ten Columbus Circle   Phone: (212) 582-1022
New York, NY 10019   Margaret E. Walsh, CAE, Exec. Dir.-Sec.
Founded: 1952. Members: 19,800. Staff: 200. State Groups: 46. Local Groups: 95. Individuals, leaders in nursing and other health professions and the community interested in solving health care problems (18,000); agencies, nursing educational institutions, and home and community health agencies (1,800). Works to assess nursing needs, improve organized nursing services and nursing education and foster collaboration between nursing and other health and community services. Provides tests used in selection of applicants to schools of nursing; also prepares tests for evaluating nursing student progress, licensing tests for state boards of nursing, and nursing service tests. Holds conferences, institutes, and workshops. Nationally accredits nursing education programs and community nursing services. Collects and disseminates data on nursing services and nursing education. Conducts studies and demonstration projects on community planning for nursing, nursing service and nursing education. Sponsors National Assembly of Constituent Leagues for Nursing; four regional assemblies; National Forum for Administrators of Nursing Services; national careers program. Bestows five awards biennially for excellence and achievement in nursing education and service. Committees: Advisory Committee on Accreditation; ANA–NLN Coordinating; Interorganization Committee with National Federation of Licensed Practical Nurses; Joint Committee–NLN and American Hospital Association of Community and Junior Colleges; Liaison Committee with National Association for Practical Nurse Education and Service; Long-Term Care; Public Affairs; Research. Councils: Associate Degree; Baccalaureate; Diploma; Home Health Agencies; Practical Nursing Programs. Divisions: Accreditation; Consultation; Continuing Education; Measurement; Public Affairs; Public Information; Research. Publications: (1) Nursing and Health Care (journal), 10/year; (2) Nursing Data Book, annual; (3) State Approved Schools of Nursing—LPN, annual; (4) State Approved Schools of Nursing—RN, annual; also publishes newsletters, memos to agency members, special interest bulletins, reports, manuals, and curriculum and evaluation guides. Formed by Merger of: Association of Collegiate Schools of Nursing, Joint Committee on Careers in Nursing, National Committee for the Improvement of Nursing

Services, National League of Nursing Education, National Nursing Accrediting Service, and National Organization for Public Health Nursing. Convention/Meeting: biennial.

SOCIETY FOR CLINICAL AND EXPERIMENTAL HYPNOSIS (SCEH)

129-A Kings Park Dr. Phone: (315) 652-7299
Liverpool, NY 13088 Marion Kenn, Adm. Dir.
Founded: 1949. Members: 950. United States division of the International Society of Hypnosis. Professional society of physicians, dentists, psychologists and certain psychiatric social workers interested in research in hypnosis and its boundary areas as well as the therapeutic use of hypnosis in clinical practice. Encourages cooperation among professional and scientific disciplines in use of hypnosis; promotes educational standards; conducts introductory and advanced workshops and continuing education seminars in therapeutic hypnosis. Gives several annual awards in recognition of outstanding contributions in the field of clinical and experimental hypnosis. Offers continuing education seminars in New York City and Chicago, IL. Committees: Advisory. Publications: (1) International Journal of Clinical and Experimental Hypnosis, quarterly; (2) Membership Directory, biennial; also publishes newletter. Affiliated with: American Association for the Advancement of Science; World Federation of Mental Health. Convention/Meeting: annual—always October. 1984 Oct. 22–27, San Antonio, TX.

SOCIETY OF NUCLEAR MEDICINE (SNM)

475 Park Ave., S. Phone: (212) 889-0717
New York, NY 10016 Henry L. Ernstthal, Exec. Dir.
Founded: 1954. Members: 9,500. Regional Groups: 16. Professional society of physicians, physicists, chemists, radiopharmacists, nuclear medicine technologists and others interested in nuclear medicine and the use of radioactive isotopes in clinical practice, research and teaching. Disseminates information concerning the utilization of nuclear phenomena in the diagnosis and treatment of disease. Offers placement bureau. Committees: Awards; Commercial Exhibits; Competence and Certification; Government Relations; Science; Socio Economics. Councils: Academic; Computer; Instrumentation; Radiopharmaceutical. Sections: Technologist. Publications: (1) Journal of Nuclear Medicine, monthly; (2) Journal of Nuclear Medicine Technology, quarterly; (3) Newsline (newsletter), quarterly; (4) Membership Directory, annual; also publishes Semiconductor Detectors in the Future of Nuclear Medicine; Nuclear Medicine in Clinical Pediatrics; Tomographic Imaging in Nuclear Medicine and other books and related materials. Convention/Meeting: annual—always June. 1984 Los Angeles, CA; 1985 Houston, TX. Technologist Section also holds a winter meeting.

WOMEN'S OCCUPATIONAL HEALTH RESOURCE CENTER (WOHRC)

School of Public Health
60 Haven Ave., B-1
Columbia University Phone: (212) 694-3464
New York, NY 10032 Jeanne M. Stellman, Ph.D., Exec. Dir.
Founded: 1978. Members: 1,000. Staff: 7. Acts as clearinghouse for women's occupational health and safety issues. Aims to increase awareness of the health and safety hazards which women face in the workplace, and to raise management awareness of the need for improved workplace and equipment design. Advises manufacturers on design standards of safety equipment. Offers technical assistance in setting up programs designed to develop

occupational health awareness; distributes questionnaires to assess occupational health and safety risks. Maintains speakers bureau. Sponsors workshops, seminars and panels on such topics as personal protective equipment, reproductive hazards, industrial safety and the hazards of household work. Maintains library with a computeriaed bibliographic information system. Publications: (1) Newsletter, bimonthly; (2) Technical Bulletin, quarterly; also publishes factsheets, illustrated fact packs and calendar.

Index